# THE JOY OF JUICING

# Gary Null, Ph.D.
## and Shelly Null

AVERY
A member of Penguin Group (USA) Inc.
New York

# THE JOY OF JUICING

*150 Imaginative, Healthful Juicing Recipes for Drinks, Soups, Salads, Sauces, Entrées, and Desserts*

**THIRD EDITION**

AVERY

Published by the Penguin Group
Penguin Group (USA) Inc., 375 Hudson Street, New York, New York 10014, USA • Penguin
Group (Canada), 90 Eglinton Avenue East, Suite 700, Toronto, Ontario M4P 2Y3, Canada (a
division of Pearson Penguin Canada Inc.) • Penguin Books Ltd, 80 Strand, London WC2R 0RL,
England • Penguin Ireland, 25 St Stephen's Green, Dublin 2, Ireland (a division of Penguin
Books Ltd) • Penguin Group (Australia), 707 Collins Street, Melbourne, Victoria 3008, Australia
(a division of Pearson Australia Group Pty Ltd) • Penguin Books India Pvt Ltd, 11 Community
Centre, Panchsheel Park, New Delhi–110 017, India • Penguin Group (NZ), 67 Apollo Drive,
Rosedale, Auckland 0632, New Zealand (a division of Pearson New Zealand Ltd) • Penguin
Books (South Africa), Rosebank Office Park, 181 Jan Smuts Avenue, Parktown North 2193,
South Africa • Penguin China, B7 Jiaming Center, 27 East Third Ring Road North, Chaoyang
District, Beijing 100020, China

Penguin Books Ltd, Registered Offices: 80 Strand, London WC2R 0RL, England

Most Avery books are available at special quantity discounts for bulk purchase for sales
promotions, premiums, fund-raising, and educational needs. Special books or book excerpts also
can be created to fit specific needs. For details, write Penguin Group (USA) Inc. Special Markets,
375 Hudson Street, New York, NY 10014.

ISBN 978-1-58333-519-2

Printed in the United States of America
10  9  8  7  6  5  4  3

BOOK DESIGN BY LOVEDOG STUDIO

While the authors have made every effort to provide accurate telephone numbers, Internet
addresses, and other contact information at the time of publication, neither the publisher nor
the authors assume any responsibility for errors, or for changes that occur after publication.
Further, the publisher does not have any control over and does not assume any responsibility
for author or third-party websites or their content.

ALWAYS LEARNING                                                              PEARSON

# Contents

# Acknowledgments

**We would like to thank** our entire New York staff for testing these recipes and Jeremy Stillman for his diligent research and editorial input.

# Introduction

**I've been juicing for myself** and others since I opened my first health food store, Creative Health Foods, in 1967. That store still stands today, but the health food store I spend most of my time in now is Gary Null's Uptown Whole Foods, at Eighty-Ninth and Broadway in Manhattan, where each day we serve fresh, organic juices to approximately two thousand customers.

Twenty years ago I wrote the first edition of *The Joy of Juicing*. It was the first of my books on the subject and became a health and nutrition bestseller. Back then I could not have imagined that today, tens of millions of individuals would be enjoying the full-spectrum benefits of fresh juice each day. Many people are now using their own extractors and blenders to make great juices and smoothies. For those who don't want to buy the produce and make it themselves, fresh bottled juices are widely available in markets across the country. Companies such as Jamba Juice have created successful business models around juicing. Even Starbucks, which recently bought out a juice bar chain, has set its sights on the fresh juice phenomenon. Who could have thought juicing would have evolved to where it is today?

Doing almost twenty hours a week of live broadcasting, all of which originates from ProgressiveRadioNetwork.com, I interview leaders in health and nutrition and field calls from listeners all over the United States and Canada. A high percentage of my guests and callers advocate juicing. More than ever, I hear testimonials of how people turned their health around while on a cleansing juice fast, or how individuals were able to lose weight or overcome conditions such as arthritis, high blood pressure, and cancer by using combinations of different juices. It's abundantly clear that increasing numbers of people are waking up to the many benefits juicing has to offer.

What you hold in your hands is the third edition of *The Joy of Juicing*. What this book contains that makes it different from previous editions and other books on this topic is a much more comprehensive understanding of what juicing can do for you. To begin with, we provide you with a guide on the basics of juicing and explain how you can get started on your own regimen today. We then take an in-depth look at the numerous scientifically established benefits of juicing. We explore the unique set of enzymes, phytonutrients, antioxidants, and chlorophylls found in nature's superfoods and how they function synergistically to enhance our well-being through cleansing and detoxification as well as rejuvenation and repair of our DNA.

Next, we bring you over one hundred juice recipes that were carefully designed to strengthen the body naturally and target specific areas of your health. Whether you are looking for a juice to help you fight off a case of the flu, improve your digestive health, or flood your body with muscle-building nutrients after an intense workout, this book is a valuable resource for individuals dealing with dozens of common ailments and those who simply want to optimize their wellness. Expanding the benefits further still, we include in our recipes a range of therapeutic vitamins, minerals, herbs, and other supplements that have been proven to promote health and healing.

Finally, we feature over one hundred delicious and creative superfood recipes. From energizing breakfast cereals, to appetizing soups and salads, to nourishing entrées and scrumptious, guilt-free desserts, these easy-to-make recipes will support your well-being and leave you satisfied.

The recipes included in this book were created with variety, taste, and therapeutic benefit in mind. But you should also understand that the recipes are intended as a starting point only. Feel free to experiment to meet your own needs and your own perception of what your body can accept. You can be as creative as you choose—and as healthy and happy as you want!

—*Gary Null*

# THE BASICS OF JUICING

# Getting Started

**You need just two basic tools** for juice and shake preparation—a quality centrifugal juicer and a workhorse blender. With an average investment of about $200, you will be set for all your juicing joys. There are a number of good juicers on the market, but make sure to pick one that has a stable motor and low heat generation. If the juicer overheats, it can kill vital enzymes and decrease the digestive value of the preparations. The stability of the mechanism is more important than the number of rpm's (revolutions per minute) the juicer boasts. The more efficiently pulp can be shredded and ejected from the unit, the less possibility there is of clogging and overheating. Also, choose a juicer that you can confidently clean with ease on a daily basis. If the thought of cleaning each time prevents you from using it, you'll never juice! A workhorse blender can be any name brand that has a good warranty policy because, if you take my advice, which I hope you will, you'll use this unit often enough to take advantage of it. Always have a backup blender or at least a backup pitcher in case of breakage. Despite the fact that they can break if dropped, I still prefer the glass blender pitchers because they are stronger and easier to clean than the plastic models.

## Go for Organic

For juicing, as for eating, you should use organically grown produce whenever possible. A fruit or vegetable that is labeled organic means that it is grown in compliance with laws certifying that the products have been grown and handled according to strict procedure without chemical input. The types of chemicals that might be used on non-organically grown produce are herbicides (weed killers), fungicides (mold killers), and insecticides. Many of these have been found to be potential cancer-causers, according to the Environmental Protection Agency. Another consideration is that pesticides and other toxins reduce a food's enzyme levels. By eating and juicing organically, you're avoiding any of those nutritional pitfalls.

What's more, organic farmers focus on maintaining healthy soil through proper tillage and crop rotation. Healthy soil contains thousands of microorganisms that help retain water and provide nutrients to the plants, nutrients that are then passed on to you. Healthy soil also produces strong, healthy plants that are better able to resist insects and disease on their own, without toxic chemicals. Because juiced produce is not cooked or boiled, it is even more important that these foods be free of toxins.

## The Way We Wash Our Produce

All fruits and vegetables should be washed properly before juicing, even organically grown produce, which does, after all, grow in dirt. If you are unable to get organically grown produce, then you must certainly wash, or in some cases peel and discard, the skin to get rid of some of the toxic chemicals. The best way to wash produce effectively is to hold it under running water while scrubbing it with a vegetable brush. Later you can use this brush to clean the stainless steel strainer found in most juicers.

## To Peel or Not to Peel

Many fruits and vegetables should be juiced with their peels on. Others, however, must be peeled because they are either too thick for the machine to grind up or have been found to contain toxic substances. Fruits that should always be peeled are kiwis, pineapples, papayas, oranges, grapefruits, tangerines, and bananas. But with oranges and grapefruits, make sure that you keep the bitter, white skin on the inside of the rind because it contains many nutrients that you do not want to lose. Watermelon rind also contains a great deal of nutrients; although it is thick, it can be juiced quite easily. (You may not want to juice the rind unless you are looking for a natural diuretic, since the juice is not as sweet as the juice of the fruit's flesh.) Waxed fruits and vegetables such as apples or turnips should always be peeled, as wax may be carcinogenic.

## Why Seeds and Pits Are the Pits

Remove all pits before juicing because they are too large and too solid to go through the juicer. Also, most seeds should be taken out because they might create an unpleasant, bitter taste. Note that apple seeds in particular *must* be removed because they have been found to contain toxic substances. Some seeds, however, such as watermelon and cantaloupe seeds, can be juiced and are in fact a dietary aid because of their natural diuretic properties, which means that they can aid the body in getting rid of excess water.

## When Raw Is a Raw Deal

Juicing vegetables raw will provide you with the maximum amount of nutrients, including life enzymes. However, a few vegetables need to be lightly steamed (and then chilled) before juicing: asparagus, broccoli, Brussels sprouts, and cauliflower. Remember to drink your juice as soon after juicing as you can, or the vitamins, minerals, and enzymes will not be as potent. However, if you juice in the morning and refrigerate the drink, it will still be fine in the evening.

## When the Blender Is Better

Juicing recipes often call for nuts, but their hard consistency makes it impossible to throw them in the juicer as is. Instead, use a blender, food processor, or food mill to grind nuts down before adding them to the rest of the juice mixture. An alternative to this is using a store-bought nut butter. Also, if a recipe calls for ice, make sure to juice the produce in the juicer and then combine it with the ice in a blender or food processor. (*Note:* Ice is never really necessary in a juice; it's fine to use water instead and have a warmer drink.) Bananas are best juiced in the blender, unless you first peel and freeze them, in which case the juicer will give you a lumpless and creamy blend.

## Protein Powder Power

You may want to add extra nutrients to your juices by mixing in some vegetable protein powder to increase not only protein content but complex carbohydrates, fiber, and vitamins and minerals as well. Protein powders can be found in health food stores and will help to complete your balanced diet. They generally consist of rice, pea, sesame seed, egg white, or soy blends. You also can add protein powder to hot cereal or use it to supplement foods on a road trip to maintain the balanced diet that often gets ignored when traveling. When you're using juice as a meal, as I often do, add two scoops of protein powder to ensure that you are not leaving out any important nutrients.

# Why Juicing?

## Antioxidants

It is well accepted that aging and degenerative diseases such as cancer, arthritis, and heart disease are the result of cellular damage brought on by free radicals, or molecules that have become unstable after losing one of their orbiting electrons. In an attempt to restore balance, a free radical will steal electrons from other molecules, causing damage through a process called oxidation. Antioxidants protect the body against excessive oxidation by neutralizing free radicals and, accordingly, play a major role in the prevention of those conditions associated with their reactions.

Free radicals are produced through normal metabolism in the body but increase with exposure to animal flesh, processed foods, alcohol, cigarettes, and radiation, as well as chemical pollutants found in water, the air, and food. Given the pervasive environmental contaminants many of us are exposed to on a daily basis, it is critically important to incorporate antioxidant-rich foods into the diet. Juicing is an ideal method of taking in high levels of these essential disease-fighting agents. The addition of antioxidant supplements to fresh juices increases their health-boosting benefits even more.

## ANTIOXIDANT SUPERSTARS

Several antioxidants stand out for their exceptional healing properties. While most of these critical nutrients are obtainable from a variety of foods, taking supplements helps ensure adequate intake. Always consult with your doctor before taking any supplements.

### Alpha-Lipoic Acid

This naturally occurring compound exhibits strong antioxidant activity in virtually every tissue in the body. In addition to protecting against oxidative stress, alpha-lipoic acid plays a key role in regulating metabolism. It also elevates glutathione levels in cells. In its reduced form, glutathione is the most potent intracellular antioxidant. Green leafy vegetables are a good source of alpha-lipoic acid.

### Bioflavonoids

Bioflavonoids are a group of water-soluble substances that help maintain the strength and proper function of the capillaries. Along with vitamin C, with which they are almost always found in food, bioflavonoids help manufacture collagen. They also protect cells against attack and invasion by viruses and bacteria. Excellent sources of bioflavonoids include grapes, rose hips, green tea, oranges, lemons, cherries, parsley, cabbage, apricots, peppers, papayas, tomatoes, broccoli, and blackberries.

### Coenzyme Q10

Every cell in the body needs coenzyme Q10 to create energy and build stamina. This critical substance converts nutrients to energy and functions as an antioxidant, helping to promote cardiovascular and muscular health. Vegetarian sources include whole grains, peanuts, spinach, and broccoli. Since levels of coenzyme Q10 decrease with age, supplementation may be especially important for people over fifty.

### Glutathione

Glutathione is a naturally occurring molecule composed of three types of amino acids: glutamate, cysteine, and glycine. Glutathione plays a central role in immune health and metabolism. The sulfur constituents found in glutathione serve as one of the body's main detoxifiers, removing poisons such as pesticides and heavy metals. Good food sources of glutathione include uncooked spinach, asparagus, garlic, avocados, bananas, and cruciferous vegetables. The production of glutathione is enhanced significantly by taking supplements such as milk thistle, N-acetyl cysteine, and alpha-lipoic acid.

### Quercetin

Quercetin stands out as a highly beneficial flavonoid antioxidant. It works as a natural antihistamine, lessening allergic reactions in a safer way than conventional drugs. Evidence suggests that quercetin has potent anti-inflammatory and anticancer properties. Onions, apples, citrus fruits, and green tea are good sources of quercetin.

### Resveratrol

This anti-inflammatory compound is one of the phytoalexins that are produced in plants during times of environmental stress, such as insect, animal, or pathogenic attack. It is a very powerful antioxidant that provides greater protection against DNA damage than even vitamin C or E. Mulberries and the skins of red grapes are particularly rich in resveratrol.

## Selenium

Selenium's primary function is as an antioxidant, protecting cells from destruction. It plays a vital role in the enzyme system and is necessary for the manufacture of prostaglandins, which control blood pressure and clotting. Selenium protects eyes against cataracts, contributes to protein production, and protects the artery walls from plaque buildup. The best vegetarian sources of selenium are Brazil nuts, mushrooms, asparagus, broccoli, onions, and tomatoes.

## Vitamin A

Vitamin A is a fat-soluble, essential vitamin necessary for bones and teeth, sperm formation, epithelial growth (skin tissue), and vision. It is essential in the maintenance of the body's immune response, which helps the body fight infections. It helps maintain healthy skin and protects the mucous membranes of the lungs, throat, mouth, and nose. It also helps the body secrete the gastric juices necessary for protein digestion and protects the linings of the digestive tract, kidneys, and bladder.

While it is abundant in carrots, especially in the form of fresh carrot juice, vitamin A is present in even higher concentrations in green leafy vegetables such as beet greens, spinach, and broccoli. Yellow or orange vegetables are also good sources.

## Vitamin C

Vitamin C has many benefits. It is an outstanding immune-system strengthener and detoxification agent. It keeps cholesterol levels down, combats stress, promotes fertility, protects against cardio-vascular disease and various forms of cancer, maintains mental health, and ultimately may prolong life. The presence of vitamin C is necessary to build collagen, the "cement" that holds together the connective tissue throughout the body. Athletes require more vitamin C for collagen synthesis and tissue repair. Vitamin C combats toxic substances in food, the air, and water and is a natural laxative. Good sources of this essential nutrient include papayas, strawberries, pineapples, kiwis, citrus fruits, sprouts, sweet potatoes, and kale. The healing capacity of vitamin C is greatly enhanced by the addition of quercetin.

### Vitamin E

Vitamin E protects our fatty acids from destruction and maintains cellular health and integrity. It is especially important for promoting the health of our muscles, cells, blood, and skin and serves as a primary defense against respiratory infection and disease. This vitamin is the major nutrient used by our bodies to protect against environmental stress. It helps dilute the harmful effects of drinking water containing lead, excess minerals such as sodium, or an otherwise unbalanced mineral content. Good sources of vitamin E include wheat germ, whole grains, unrefined cereals, seeds, nuts, organic eggs, and leafy greens eaten with cold-pressed oils.

The active chemical ingredient in vitamin E is pure alpha-tocopherol. If you're seeking a supplement, get natural vitamin E. Research indicates that the natural form is more active and therefore more useful than the synthetic variety.

### Zinc

Like selenium, zinc is a mineral that displays antioxidant properties. Zinc feeds over one hundred enzyme systems in the brain as well as various systems throughout the body. Zinc helps combat viruses and bacteria and is essential in the formation of stomach acid; without sufficient zinc, malabsorption syndrome occurs. Vegetarian sources of zinc include wheat germ, tahini, pumpkin seeds, and sunflower seeds. Supplementing may be especially helpful for people over fifty, who are commonly deficient in zinc.

## Chlorophyll

Giving plants their green color is a natural compound known as chlorophyll. Utilizing light energy to convert water and carbon dioxide to glucose, chlorophyll plays a vital role in plant energy production. Research has found that this substance not only sustains plant life but has profoundly beneficial effects on human health as well.

The molecular structure of chlorophyll is very similar to that of hemoglobin, the substance that transports oxygen in the bloodstream. Consuming chlorophyll-rich fruits and vegetables improves the efficiency of oxygen transport in the body, which works to thin the blood and, in turn, helps prevent clotting and heart disease. Taking chlorophyll enhances any exercise program because the body requires oxygen to develop muscles and burn fat.

Chlorophyll exhibits strong anti-inflammatory and anti-viral activity and serves as an effective chelation agent, removing toxic heavy metals such as mercury from the body. Studies have observed the ability of this substance to aid in the prevention and treatment of cancer. Due to its antibacterial properties, many individuals with bad breath and body odor use chlorophyll mouthwashes or baths for relief.

As with other beneficial nutrients found in whole foods, juicing maximizes the absorption of chlorophyll. Some of the best sources of this rejuvenating substance include asparagus, barley grass, broccoli, chlorella, collard greens, kale, leeks, parsley, spirulina, and wheatgrass.

## Detoxification

Toxic substances abound in our air, water, soil, and food. A healthy person can often eliminate harmful substances through the liver and other organs. On the other hand, an individual whose health is compromised, or on a diet too high in fats, processed proteins, sodium, refined sugars, and other refined foods, has a reduced capacity to rid the body of toxins. When this happens, the toxins accumulate.

The buildup of toxins can severely depress the immune system. In the past half-century, with the increase in environmental pollution and dependence on processed foods, we have witnessed higher rates of diseases such as cancer, heart disease, and arthritis. People in polluted urban or suburban areas may say they have little control over toxic exposure, but there are things we all can do. We can stop smoking, drinking alcohol, using drugs, and consuming processed foods. We can begin to eat fresh, untreated, raw foods and fresh juices, whose detoxifying nutrients are more available to the body than those in packaged foods.

Toxins in foods may not all be poisons in the classic sense. They often do their damage more insidiously by inhibiting the actions of enzymes. Enzymes are important activators of almost every digestive or energy-producing activity in the body. Many things can go wrong if enzymes don't do their work properly. Our digestive systems can become sluggish and slow down, causing fat digestion to become difficult and protein digestion to be inefficient. Our kidneys and liver then become overloaded and fat may be deposited in our arteries. Cardiovascular and other degenerative diseases can result.

Foods that are commercially fertilized may also be denuded of their proper mineral levels. For example, potassium—the most important activator of enzymes in the body—is one of the most vital minerals to be lost in this way. Without the right amount of potassium, the natural chemicals and enzymes that make digestion efficient could not function, yet potassium is reduced—and sodium added—in many of our processed foods. Toxins deplete the body's potassium stores further still, changing our basic metabolic balance and opening the door for a host of potential health complications. The detoxification process will often depend on rebuilding potassium supplies in the body by including fresh fruits and vegetables in the daily diet. Drinking juices that contain potassium-rich foods such as Swiss chard, potatoes, papayas, avocados, and bananas can be a good way to jump-start this process.

The key to detoxification is offering the body the right nutrients. Allow the body to open up the eliminative processes, in which the liver and digestive tract play key roles. Start to detoxify by getting used to natural juices, natural mineral sources, and other organic substances. This process may be a slow one at the start. When toxins have had so long to build up, their breakdown also will take time.

## Enzymes

Enzymes are natural substances that stimulate some of the internal reactions necessary for life. Our bodies contain more than seven hundred types of enzymes, each one responsible for a different task. A shortage of even one type can dramatically affect health. Enzymes are found throughout the body, with the most vital ones in the salivary glands, pancreas, stomach walls, intestines, and liver.

Without enzymes, food could not be digested. Enzymes help transform food products into muscles, nerves, bones, and glands. They assist in storing excess nutrients in the muscles and liver for future access, help create urea to be excreted in the urine, and facilitate the departure of carbon dioxide from the lungs. Enzymes also help stop bleeding and serve to decompose poisonous hydrogen peroxide to liberate needed oxygen. They help us breathe and attack poisons in the blood.

Mental strain or worry has a deleterious effect on enzyme actions. It is better to avoid large meals during such times, since stressful situations tend to inhibit the flow of enzymes and interfere with the actions of the digestive tract. To perform their life-sustaining tasks, enzymes must be continually replaced. Unnatural environmental components such as pollution, food additives, and stress all negatively affect the makeup of cells and increase the need for health-promoting enzymes.

Enzymes are abundant in fresh raw foods, especially fruits and vegetables. They cannot, however, survive at temperature higher than 122 degrees Fahrenheit, which means that they won't exist in cooked foods. The absorption of enzymes depends on how food is broken down. Food that is not chewed well enters the digestive canal only partially prepared, and, as a result, enzymes are not fully assimilated.

It is interesting to note that in Asian cultures, even though food is an important social focal point, most people remain naturally slim. That's because the traditional Asian diet consists mostly of fresh, raw fruits and vegetables, lightly cooked fare, fermented foods, and rice—all enzyme-rich choices.

Here in the West, though, our diets can be enzyme-poor because enzymes are largely destroyed by the heat of cooking and processing things, which we do a lot of in our culture. Juicing, on the other hand, keeps produce enzyme-rich. When the juice is consumed promptly or after a brief period of storage in the freezer or a vacuum bottle, you will benefit from the enzymes.

Following is a list of some of the enzymes that function as digestive aids and the foods that contain them. Juicing and eating these foods may help to prevent or overcome overweight conditions:

* Bromelain, found in pineapples
* Esterase, found in many plant foods (starchy vegetables, such as potatoes, and leafy vegetables, such as lettuce)

* Hemicellulase, found in seeds and green plants (spinach, lettuce, arugula, broccoli, cauliflower, kale, Swiss chard, and parsley)
* Invertase, found in cucumbers and green plants
* Lactase, found in tomatoes, persimmons, apples, and peaches
* Lipase, found in green plants, wheat germ, and flaxseed
* Maltase, found in beet leaves, green plants, bananas, and mushrooms
* Nuclease, found in mung beans
* Papain, found in papayas
* Sucrase, found in green plants, beet leaves and stems, and bananas

## Phytonutrients

Plant-based foods also contain a vast range of ingredients known as phytonutrients or phytochemicals. (*Phyto* simply means "plant.") Phytonutrients are chemicals produced by plants to help withstand the damaging effects of ultraviolet light, freezing, drought, parasites, and other dangers. A single fruit or vegetable may contain up to several hundred phytochemicals, many of which have been proven to promote health.

Phytonutrients express themselves as rainbow colors, and we get the most benefit from eating a variety of these pigments. For example, studies have shown that lycopene, the red phytochemical found in tomatoes, beets, and watermelon, contributes to heart health; indoles, found in broccoli, kale, Brussels sprouts, and other cruciferous vegetables, possess anticancer properties. Citrus fruits contain phytochemicals known as terpenes, which boost eye health and help protect against dental decay and ulcers.

There is still much to learn regarding the value of specific plant chemicals, as well as the effects of phytonutrients working together. From a scientific standpoint, we may never comprehend the full benefit derived from combined phytonutrients, but we are learning that nature, in its wisdom, has combined ingredients that complement one another and work synergistically. Thus in the health field we have the saying, "The whole food is greater than the sum of its parts." And for speedy healing and overall well-being, juicing is better yet.

# Superfoods

**Superfoods are those fruits, vegetables,** nuts, legumes, seeds, herbs, and spices that possess extraordinary healing properties. These nutritional all-stars are an outstanding source of nature's most powerful antioxidants, vitamins, minerals, enzymes, chlorophyll, and phytonutrients. Juicing superfoods is the best way to flood your body with their life-sustaining nutrients.

## Vegetables

### Beets

Drink beet juice to nourish the liver, one of the most important organs of the body with hundreds of different functions. If your liver is functioning well, most likely everything else in your body is, too. Furthermore, beet juice cleanses the blood and relieves high blood pressure.

### Cabbage

Cabbage is high in vitamin K and cancer-fighting substances known as indoles. Drinking cabbage juice is an effective means of alleviating stomach ailments such as peptic ulcers. Packed with antioxidants called anthocyanins, red cabbage is a powerful anti-inflammatory food.

### Carrots

The bright orange color of carrots is your first clue that this sweet, crunchy vegetable is packed with protective, disease-fighting antioxidant compounds. One cup of raw carrots has just 54 calories and provides an astounding 683 percent of the recommended daily value of vitamin A and 221 percent of the RDV of vitamin K. Carrots contain carotenoids, natural fat-soluble pigments found in certain plants that provide their bright coloration and serve as antioxidants and a source for vitamin A activity. These carotenoids are associated with protection from heart disease and cancer, improved night vision, and improved blood sugar regulation.

### Celery

Celery has a cleansing diuretic effect, whether it is taken as a tea or as a juice. Celery's alkalinity also makes it soothing to the digestive system. The natural sodium in celery promotes good cell chemistry.

### Collard Greens

Chock-full of vitamin K, vitamin A, calcium, and powerful detoxifying phytonutrients, collard greens are true nutritional powerhouses. Collard greens are abundant in glucosinolates, which are phytochemicals that play a key role in detoxification. This cruciferous family vegetable is also a good source of indole compounds and alpha-linolenic acid (ALA), making it a great addition to any anti-inflammatory diet.

### Cucumbers

Cucumbers are a wonderful source of hydration and restorative phytonutrients. They contain significant amounts of vitamin C, vitamin K, and potassium, as well as silica, a compound needed for healthy connective tissue. Researchers are currently looking into the potential anticancer properties of cucurbitacins, a phytonutrient abundant in cucumbers.

### Kale

Kale may be one of the healthiest greens for your bones. Just one cup of cooked kale contains over 1,300 percent of the recommended daily value of vitamin K. Kale is also high in calcium and is a good source of manganese, which helps promote bone density. Kale is the top leafy green source of free radical scavenging carotenoids.

### Sea Vegetables

Sea vegetables, such as sea palm, nori, kelp, wakame, and dulse, are available in natural food and Asian markets. They are loaded with minerals, especially iodine, which is important for thyroid function and something we often don't get enough of. Sea vegetables also provide a good amount of magnesium and calcium.

### Spinach

High amounts of vitamin A, vitamin K, calcium, magnesium, and numerous other nutrients make the nutritional profile of spinach impressive. Similar to other leafy greens, spinach is a good source of lutein and zeaxanthin, phytonutrients that help protect against macular degeneration, a cause of blindness. Research shows the anticancer and anti-inflammatory properties of this common vegetable.

### Wheatgrass

A great source of chlorophyll, vitamins, minerals, and amino acids, wheatgrass offers a myriad of benefits. The high chlorophyll content in wheatgrass makes it a superb detoxifier and anticancer superfood. Wheatgrass is also rich in immune-enhancing antioxidants such as vitamins A, C, and E, as well as zinc. Research suggests that wheatgrass may help curb inflammatory conditions such as ulcerative colitis.

Wheatgrass can be juiced by using a wheatgrass press. You can also make wheatgrass juice by squeezing the grass into clusters with your hands and juicing these clusters through a traditional fruit and vegetable juicer.

## Fruits

### Apples

Fresh apple juice helps to correct skin and liver disorders. It has a laxative effect and is a valuable aid to digestion and weight loss. Apples contain the flavonoid called quercetin, which acts as a natural antihistamine and anti-inflammatory. Make sure to juice the skin of apples because it is packed with free radical scavenging polyphenol antioxidants.

### Bananas

Bananas are a great source of vitamin $B_6$, manganese, and potassium. They also contain pectin, a soluble fiber that absorbs fluid, helping to normalize movement through the digestive tract and improve nutrient absorption. In addition, bananas are rich in a probiotic compound called fructooligosaccharide, which may specifically aid in calcium absorption by stimulating the production of probiotic bacteria in the colon. Increased probiotic bacteria also help protect the body against harmful microorganisms that can cause digestive problems and other ailments.

### Blueberries

Blueberries contain an impressive array of antioxidants that have been shown in studies to support health in numerous ways. These fruits are particularly rich in a class of phytonutrients known as anthocyanidins, which give blueberries their blue-red pigment. Anthocyanidins are credited with enhancing the effects of vitamin C, promoting heart health, and protecting the brain from oxidative stress. Another antioxidant found in blueberries is ellagic acid, which research indicates can help reverse cancer.

### Grapefruits

Vitamin C, pectin, and a host of other beneficial nutrients are found in grapefruits. They are rich in carotenoid antioxidants, such as lycopene, which have been observed in studies to curb oxidative stress and combat cancer. Grapefruits are also high in phytochemicals called limonoids. Preliminary research indicates these compounds exhibit strong anticarcinogenic activity.

### Kiwis

Aside from being a great source of vitamin C, kiwis are rich in several classes of antioxidants including carotenoids and flavonoids. The scientific literature demonstrates the efficacy of kiwis in protecting heart health and inhibiting respiratory ailments such as asthma. The seeds of kiwis contain alpha-linolenic acid (ALA), a type of omega-3 fatty acid that fights oxidative stress.

### Lemons

The large quantities of vitamin C and citric acid found in lemons support immune system function and can help stave off the formation of painful kidney stones. In addition, lemons are among the most alkaline-forming foods, meaning they help the body maintain a blood pH level in its ideal range of 7.2 to 7.4, which is important for the prevention and treatment of cancer and other diseases.

### Melons

Melon juices are wonderful kidney cleansers and are highly alkalinizing. Be sure to juice the rind; it provides a wide range of enzymes, minerals, and chlorophyll.

### Oranges

One orange contains only 62 calories and is packed with vitamin C, folate, and significant amounts of vitamin $B_1$, potassium, vitamin A, and calcium. Like blueberries, the orange's vibrant color is indicative of its potent antioxidants. While oranges are loaded with antioxidants, it is the hesperidin flavonoid that stands out for its strong anti-inflammatory properties. Besides acting to promote healthy blood vessel function, hesperidin is also beneficial in reducing cholesterol. Most of this phytonutrient content is found in the peel of the orange.

### Papayas

High concentrations of inflammation-fighting carotenoids give papaya its deep orange hue. This tropical fruit is abundant in vitamin C and anticancer compounds like lycopene and isothiocyanates. Papayas also have proteolytic enzymes that promote digestion, boost immunity, and help heal body tissue.

### Pineapples

Pineapples contain high amounts of bromelain, a type of enzyme that has been shown to shield against several chronic diseases. Research demonstrates the ability of bromelain to aid digestion, ease inflammation, and mitigate the symptoms of arthritis. Additionally, pineapples pack a large dose of vitamin C, vitamin $B_1$, and manganese. Juicing pineapples is a great way to easily absorb these essential compounds.

### Strawberries

Bursting with vitamins, minerals, and free radical scavenging flavonoids and polyphenols, strawberries are an immensely healthful fruit. The consumption of strawberries is linked with healthy cholesterol levels and reduced inflammation. Strawberries have also been shown to help prevent the spread of cancer.

## Nuts, Seeds, Beans, and Legumes

### Almonds

Aside from their high protein content, almonds have an abundance of health-boosting vitamins and minerals including vitamin E, folic acid, magnesium, potassium, and selenium. Mixing a few tablespoons of almond butter into a smoothie is a delicious way of obtaining important nutrients.

### Carob

A type of legume, carob is a rich-tasting dark brown powder made from the dried pods of a Mediterranean evergreen tree. Carob is high in antioxidant tannins, calcium, and dietary fiber. Carob powder is naturally sweet and can be used as a healthful alternative to chocolate.

### Cashews

Packed with heart-healthy monounsaturated fat and essential minerals like magnesium, copper, and phosphorus, cashews are a nutritive and versatile food that can be easily incorporated into smoothies in the form of cashew butter.

### Flaxseeds

In addition to their high dietary fiber content, flaxseeds have high levels of anti-inflammatory omega-3 fatty acids such as alpha-linolenic acid (ALA). Flaxseeds are also by far nature's best source of lignans, which are polyphenol antioxidants that promote cardiovascular health. Taking flaxseed oil or grinding flaxseeds before eating them ensures maximum absorption of omega-3s.

### Macadamia Nuts

Macadamia nuts are abundant in an array of beneficial constituents including vitamin E, several B vitamins, and omega-3 fatty acids. Macadamias are notable for their ability to decrease the risk of cardiovascular disease and inflammatory markers. The high fiber content in macadamia nuts promotes digestion and satiety.

### Peanuts

Peanuts, though commonly grouped with seeds and nuts, are actually members of the legume family. Their high protein content is well known, but peanuts are also a good source of vitamin $B_3$, copper, manganese, coenzyme Q10, and vitamin E. Research demonstrates the ability of this staple of the American diet to lower the risk of cardiovascular illness. A scoop of peanut butter imparts a wholesome creaminess to any smoothie. Be sure to use an organic variety that does not contain additives.

### Sesame Seeds

Obtained from the sesame plant, these seeds are an excellent source of protein, unsaturated fatty acids, calcium, magnesium, niacin, and vitamins A and E. Try them in the form of tahini paste, which is made by grinding hulled, unroasted sesame seeds.

### Soybeans

Whether in the form of tofu, soy milk, miso, or tempeh, soybeans are a versatile and highly nutritious food. A one-cup serving of cooked soybeans has 300 calories and packs a whopping 29 grams of protein. Soy contains tryptophan, an amino acid that occurs in proteins and is essential for growth and normal metabolism. Tryptophan is a precursor of niacin, which helps the body produce serotonin, a chemical that acts as a calming agent in the brain and plays a role in sleep regulation. Soy also offers high concentrations of molybdenum, a trace mineral that plays a role in three enzyme systems involved in the metabolism of carbohydrates, fats, and proteins and is also found in tooth enamel. Because soybeans are a good source of protein, iron, and essential omega-3 fatty acids, they make excellent replacements for meat.

### Sunflower Seeds

Sunflower seeds are sun-energized, nutritional powerhouses rich in protein (about 30 percent), calcium, phosphorus, magnesium, zinc, and vitamin D (one of the few vegetable sources of this vitamin). Their high mineral content is the result of the sunflower's extensive root system, which penetrates deep into the subsoil seeking nutrients. Sunflower butter added to smoothies enhances both taste and nutritional value.

## Herbs and Spices

### Aloe Vera

Widely known as a soothing topical treatment for sunburns and wounds, this herb also offers a number of benefits when taken orally. It is antiseptic, antimicrobial, and anti-inflammatory and supplies the system with amino acids, vitamins, and minerals such as calcium, copper, iron, phosphorus, potassium, and zinc. Aloe vera contains live enzymes, including amylase, lactic dehydrogenase, and lipase, as well as the essential fatty acids needed for optimum health.

### Ashwagandha

Ashwagandha is a popular remedy used in Ayurvedic medicine to treat a long list of ailments. Studies indicate that this herb may significantly reduce stress on the nervous system and help protect against neurodegenerative illnesses such as Alzheimer's disease. In addition, ashwagandha has been observed to combat anxiety and inhibit cancer growth.

### Astragalus

Although new to the West, astragalus is a time-honored Chinese remedy. In fact, traditional Chinese medicine texts from four thousand years ago says astragalus has the ability to strengthen resistance to disease. Modern science now confirms these claims, demonstrating that cells damaged by cancer and radiation are stimulated to full function with the introduction of this herb. Taking astragalus is an excellent way to enhance the immune system.

### Cayenne

Cayenne helps the body metabolize cholesterol and promotes circulation. Chili peppers and other spicy foods act as expectorants in the bronchial passages, benefitting patients with chronic bronchitis and emphysema. Surprisingly, the capsaicin that stings your mouth in food is also an effective pain suppressant, inhibiting the relay of pain signals to the central nervous system. Finally, chili peppers have an effect on the brain: the burning they cause in the mouth provokes the release of endorphins, the body's natural morphine that blocks pain and induces a sensation of pleasure related to "runner's high." For a heart-healthy jolt to your juices, add ⅛–½ teaspoon of cayenne pepper.

### Cinnamon

Cinnamon possesses several remarkable medicinal qualities; it is antibacterial and antifungal and acts as a blood thinner. Cinnamon is also a very effective diarrhea remedy. The high antioxidant activity in cinnamon makes it an excellent anti-inflammatory spice.

### Evening Primrose

The oil derived from the North American evening primrose plant supplies the body with a healthful dose of essential fatty acids. Evening primrose oil may provide significant relief to individuals suffering from a wide range of ailments including diabetes, premenstrual syndrome, and skin disorders.

### Garlic

Garlic's distinctive odor is due to its sulfur-containing compounds—the most important being allicin—which also are responsible for many of its therapeutic effects. Allicin is a powerful inhibitor of bacterial growth with an extremely broad spectrum; hundreds of studies have confirmed its effectiveness fighting off as many as seventy-two separate infectious agents. The scientific literature demonstrates that garlic lowers cholesterol and thins the blood, lowering the chances of dangerous blood clots, and possesses strong anticancer properties. In addition, garlic is an effective decongestant for common colds and can prevent or ease chronic bronchitis.

The best way to get garlic is to grow your own or buy bulbs that are as fresh as possible. Raw garlic is most effective, especially in antibacterial activity, but garlic in cooking retains many of its therapeutic benefits. A teaspoon or two of freshly chopped garlic is a healthful addition to all menus. Juicing with garlic maximizes the bioavailability of its beneficial constituents.

### Ginger

This versatile root reduces blood pressure and cholesterol and stimulates the heart. Ginger is a more powerful anticoagulant than garlic or onions. Gingerols—a group of powerful antioxidants unique to ginger—have been shown to fight inflammation, viruses, and parasites, as well as destroy cancer cells. It is also useful for upset stomachs and motion sickness. Adding one ounce of fresh ginger to a juice is an excellent way to take advantage of this food's healing properties.

### Ginkgo Biloba

The ginkgo tree has survived for hundreds of thousands of years due to its powerful immune system. An extract of the leaf of the tree has been found to support human health in numerous ways. This plant improves circulation to the microcapillaries of the brain and heart so that needed nutrients and oxygen can get to all the tissues. Supplementing with ginkgo biloba is associated with improvement in mental function and mood enhancement, as well as relief from inflammatory conditions such as arthritis.

### Ginseng

This herb is considered the master herb by the Chinese, and research demonstrates that it improves physical efficiency and stamina, pulls heavy metals such as mercury, lead, and cadmium out of tissues, and enhances mental concentration. Both panax and Siberian ginseng are adaptogens, or substances that serve as balancing mechanisms in the body. Adaptogens raise low blood pressure but also bring high blood pressure down, for example. An adaptogen has nonspecific properties that enable animals to cope with both physical and mental stress more efficiently, to be more resilient, and to maintain a balance, or homeostasis, under widely varying conditions. As an adaptogen, ginseng helps the body to balance itself under a variety of stress factors.

### Green Tea

Green tea is an outstanding source of healing antioxidants; there are eight to ten times as many polyphenols in green tea as there are in fruits and vegetables. The phytochemicals in green tea and green tea extract have been shown in studies to counter many ailments, including cancer, arthritis, and cardiovascular disease.

### Maca

An oily root vegetable native to South America, maca is rapidly growing in popularity due to its remarkable health benefits. This adaptogen packs a large dose of vitamins, minerals, uncommon phytonutrients, and healthy fatty acids that combine to boost energy and support the immune and endocrine systems.

### Medicinal Mushrooms

Reishi mushrooms help reduce anxiety, hypertension, and high cholesterol and stimulate the immune system. In addition to fighting fatigue, cordyceps mushrooms display anti-inflammatory and anticancer properties. Shiitake mushrooms contain lentinan, an immune modular that can help lessen the effects of chemotherapy and combat several forms of cancer.

### Milk Thistle

The milk thistle herb offers strong protection to the liver, helping it release accumulated toxins and cleanse the body. This herb contains compounds called silibinins, which the scientific literature suggests may be helpful as a complementary treatment for cancer, diabetes, and cardiovascular disease.

### Rhodiola

An adaptogenic herb that has been used as a remedy for thousands of years in Europe and Asia, rhodiola is commonly used by alternative health practitioners to treat aging-related diseases as well as low energy and stress.

### Turmeric

A relative of ginger root, turmeric is an exceptional superfood spice. Its main active component, curcumin, is a powerful antioxidant that produces a favorable effect on no fewer than ten causative factors in cancer development. Studies reveal that turmeric can effectively inhibit inflammatory conditions such as ulcerative colitis and rheumatoid arthritis.

# JUICES AND SMOOTHIES

What follows is my own collection of unique juice and smoothie recipes. Not only do these beverages taste great, but they offer a broad spectrum of nutritional benefits. To each recipe we have also added vitamins, minerals, herbs, and other supplements that have been shown by modern science to support physical well-being in many powerful ways. These recipes are not intended to treat any medical condition or serve as a substitute for professional medical care; they are merely suggestions to enhance the body's overall health. Always consult with your physician before taking any supplements.

# Allergies

## Allergy Relief Blend

4 cups strawberries, hulled and halved

1 cup pineapple, rind removed, cored and cubed

1 medium papaya, peeled, pitted, and cubed

100 mg grape seed extract

10,000 IU vitamin A

1. Push the strawberries, pineapple, and papaya through the juicer.

2. Stir in the grape seed extract and vitamin A.

3. Pour over ice, and serve immediately.

*Makes 2½–3 Cups*

# Antihistamine Supreme

8 large apples, cored and quartered

8 large pears, cored and quartered

4 ounces fresh ginger root, sliced into ½-inch pieces

800 mg quercetin

200 mg bromelain

5,000 mg vitamin C

2 cups sparkling mineral water

16–20 ice cubes

1.  Push the apples, pears, and ginger through the juicer.

2.  In a large pitcher, combine the juice mixture with the quercetin, bromelain, vitamin C, and mineral water. Stir together until well combined.

3.  Pour into glasses filled with ice and serve immediately.

*Makes 11 Cups*

# Dandelion Fix

2 apples, cored and quartered

3 cups honeydew melon, cubed, rind removed

1 tablespoon honey

1 cup chopped dandelion greens

1 cup chopped broccoli

1-inch piece ginger root

100 mg pycnogenol

1.  Push all the ingredients except the pycnogenol through the juicer and stir well.

2.  Stir in the pycnogenol.

3.  Chill before serving.

*Makes 2 Cups*

# Sneeze Ease

½ medium cantaloupe, cubed, rind removed

½ small watermelon, cubed, rind removed

1 medium lemon, peeled and quartered

2 cups raspberries

1,000 mg vitamin C powder

75 mg butterbur extract

1. Push the melons and lemon through the juicer.

2. Blend the raspberries, vitamin C, and butterbur extract with the juice mixture in a blender.

3. Serve immediately.

*Makes 2–2½ Cups*

# Anti-aging

## Anti-inflammation Libation

3 tablespoons flaxseeds

½ cup rolled oats

1 medium apple, peeled, cored, and quartered

1 medium peach, peeled, pitted, and quartered

2 cups vanilla-flavored rice milk

2 tablespoons carob powder

250 mg alpha-lipoic acid

400 mg curcumin

1. In a grinder, grind the flaxseeds to a very fine consistency.

2. Separately grind the oats to a very fine consistency.

3. Blend the fruit, rice milk, carob powder, alpha-lipoic acid, and curcumin with the ground oats and flaxseeds until smooth.

4. Serve immediately.

*Makes 3–4 Cups*

# Antioxidant Punch

½ cup honeydew melon, cubed, with rind on

15 grapes with seeds, any color

¼ cup coconut water

2 tablespoons aloe vera concentrate

500 mg American ginseng

120 mg ginkgo biloba extract

1. Push the honeydew melon and grapes through the juicer.

2. Add the coconut water, aloe vera concentrate, ginseng, and ginkgo biloba to the juice mixture and stir well.

3. Serve immediately.

*Makes 1–1½ Cups*

# Citrus Strength Supreme

8 large grapefruits, peeled and cubed

12 large oranges, peeled and cubed

8 large limes, peeled and quartered

4 large lemons, peeled and quartered

1,000 mg rhodiola root extract

250 mg ashwagandha extract

16–20 ice cubes

1. Push the grapefruits, oranges, limes, and lemons through the juicer. Stir the juice well.

2. Stir in the rhodiola root extract and ashwagandha extract.

3. Pour into glasses filled with ice and serve immediately.

*Makes 12 Cups*

# Fountain of Youth

1 cup green grapes with seeds

1 cup purple grapes with seeds

½ cantaloupe, cubed, rind removed

2 medium zucchini, sliced

1 medium tomato, quartered

2 tablespoons vegetarian protein powder

500 mg wild blueberry extract

1. Push all the fruits and vegetables through the juicer.

2. Add the protein powder and wild blueberry extract to the juice mixture and stir well.

3. Serve immediately.

*Makes 2–3 Cups*

# Tasty Rejuvenation

24 large peaches, peeled, pitted, and quartered
    (about 12 cups)

½ large pineapple, rind removed, cored and cut
    into 1-inch cubes (about 4 cups)

2 lemons, peeled and quartered

2 limes, peeled and quartered

1 cup basil

4 cups frozen pitted cherries

4 peeled bananas, frozen

1 tablespoon turmeric

16–20 ice cubes

1. Push the peaches, pineapple, lemons, limes, and basil through the juicer.

2. Blend the cherries, bananas, turmeric, and ice with the juice mixture in a blender on high speed until smooth.

3. Serve immediately.

*Makes 1½ Gallons*

# Tropical Energy

2 medium guavas, peeled, seeded, and quartered
   lengthwise
2 small cucumbers, quartered lengthwise
1 orange, peeled and quartered
300 mg boswellia
500 mg astragalus

1. Push the guavas, cucumbers, and orange through the juicer in the order listed. Stir the juice well.

2. Stir in the boswellia and astragalus.

3. Serve immediately.

*Makes 1–1½ Cups*

# Vibrance Elixir

2 pineapples, rind removed, cored and cut into
  1-inch cubes

4 large limes, peeled and quartered

2 cups unsweetened cranberry juice

1 cup Concord grape juice

2,500 mg vitamin C

2,000 IU vitamin E

24 ice cubes

1. Push the pineapples and limes through the juicer.

2. In a large pitcher or punch bowl, combine the juice mixture, cranberry juice, grape juice, vitamin C, vitamin E, and ice. Stir together until well combined.

3. Serve immediately.

*Makes 8 Cups*


# Well-Being Wellspring

1-inch piece ginger root

1 medium pineapple, rind removed, cored and cubed

3 peeled bananas, frozen

½ cup fennel flowers and stems

1 medium passion fruit

½ teaspoon cayenne pepper

1 tablespoon raw maca powder

1. Push the ginger and pineapple through the juicer.

2. Blend the remaining ingredients with the juice mixture in a blender until smooth.

3. Pour over ice and serve immediately.

*Makes 3–3½ Cups*

# Arthritis

## Anti-inflame Sprout Power

    1 cup sunflower sprouts

    1 cup buckwheat sprouts

    1 cup alfalfa sprouts

    4–5 medium radishes

    1 bunch kale, chopped

    3 medium apples, cored and quartered

    2 ounces wheatgrass juice

    400 mg glucosamine sulfate

    400 mg chondroitin sulfate

1. Push all of the sprouts, the radishes, kale, and apples through the juicer.

2. Add the wheatgrass juice, glucosamine, and chondroitin to the juice mixture and stir well.

3. Serve immediately.

*Makes 3 Cups*

# Gout Fighter

    1 cup strawberries, hulled

    1 cup pitted cherries

    1 medium slice cantaloupe, rind removed

    1,000 mg methylsulfonylmethane (MSM)

    3–4 ounces mineral water

    5–6 ice cubes

1.  Blend all the ingredients together in a blender until smooth.

2.  Serve immediately.

*Makes 3 Cups*


# Joint Strength

    ½ small head cabbage, any color, chopped

    2 oranges, peeled and quartered

    ¼ cup chopped broccoli

    1 cup chopped endive

    2 apples, cored and quartered

    200 mg decursinol

    50 mg hyaluronic acid

1.  Push the cabbage, oranges, broccoli, endive, and apples through the juicer in the order listed.

2.  Stir in the decursinol and hyaluronic acid.

3.  Serve immediately.

*Makes 3 Cups*

# Max Mobility

3 carrots, peeled, sliced lengthwise, tops removed

2 apples, cored and quartered

½ cup non-flavored soy milk

1,000 mg methylsulfonylmethane (MSM)

400 mg curcumin

1. Push the carrots and apples through the juicer.

2. Add the soy milk, MSM, and curcumin to the carrot juice and stir well.

3. Serve immediately.

*Makes About 2 Cups*

# Old Man Arthritis

1 large yam, quartered

1 cup pineapple, rind removed, cored and cubed

1 large orange, peeled and quartered

1 cup chopped kale

½ cup chopped walnuts

100 mg boswellia

2,000 mcg vitamin K

1. Push the yams, pineapple, orange, and kale through the juicer.

2. Blend the walnuts, boswellia, and vitamin K with the juice mixture in a blender until the liquid thickens.

3. Serve immediately.

*Makes 3 Cups*

# Brain and Nervous System Health

## Brain Power

12 lychee nuts, pitted, skins removed

2 oranges, peeled and quartered

2 mangoes, peeled, pitted, and diced

100 mg Korean ginseng

100 mg ginkgo biloba

1. Push the lychee nuts, oranges, and mangoes through the juicer.

2. Blend the ginseng and ginkgo biloba with the juice mixture in a blender.

3. Serve immediately.

*Makes 1½– 2 Cups*

# Cerebral Tonic

1½ cups green beans

½ head organic cabbage, shredded

2 cups chopped collard greens

1 cup chopped spinach

2 medium peaches, pitted and quartered

3 oranges, peeled and quartered

200 mcg selenium

40 mg zinc picolinate

1. Push all the vegetables and fruits through the juicer.

2. Stir in the selenium and zinc picolinate.

3. Serve immediately.

*Makes 3–4 Cups*

# Cognition Cocktail

1 large yam, quartered

3 oranges or grapefruits, peeled and quartered

125 mg ashwagandha extract

1. Push the yam and oranges or grapefruits through juicer. Stir juice well.

2. Stir in the ashwagandha extract.

3. Serve immediately.

*Makes 2 Cups*

# Head Cleaner

  1 onion, peeled and quartered

  3 cloves garlic, peeled

  2 celery stalks

  ½-inch piece ginger root

  1 turnip, halved

  3 tablespoons honey

  One standard serving of vitamin B complex (containing
    at least 800 mcg folic acid)

  50 mg DHEA

1. Push the onion, garlic, celery, ginger, and turnip through the juicer.

2. Add the honey, vitamin B complex, and DHEA to the juice mixture and stir well.

3. Serve immediately.

*Makes 1–1½ Cups*


# Inner Clear

  ½ medium organic garlic bulb, peeled

  1 cup cranberries

  ½ small onion, peeled and quartered

  1 cup collard greens

  1 cup blackberries

  3 tablespoons raw honey

  ½ cup plain soy yogurt

  500 IU vitamin E

1. Push the garlic, cranberries, onion, collard greens, and blackberries through the juicer.

2. Blend the raw honey, soy yogurt, and vitamin E with the juice mixture until smooth.

3. Serve immediately.

*Makes 1½–2 Cups*

# Cancer

## Berry Cream Boost

1 cup blackberries

1 cup strawberries, hulled

½ cup cranberries

1 cup coconut milk

¼ cup soy milk

½ teaspoon vanilla extract

1 tablespoon protein powder

250 mg Korean ginseng

450 mg astragalus

1. Blend all the ingredients together in a blender.

2. Serve immediately.

*Makes 2½–3 Cups*

# Black and Blue Nutrient Shake

¼ cup blueberries

¼ cup blackberries

¼ cup black currants

2 tablespoons protein powder

2 tablespoons green powder

¼ teaspoon ginseng

1. Blend all the ingredients together in a blender until smooth.

2. Serve immediately.

*Makes 1–1½ Cups*

# Immunity Punch

1 honeydew melon, rind removed, seeded and cut into
    2-inch pieces (about 8 cups)

4 large oranges, peeled and quartered

4 large limes, peeled and quartered

2 large grapefruits, peeled and quartered

2 large lemons, peeled and quartered

4 mangoes, peeled, pitted, and cut into 2-inch pieces

1 cup blueberries

20–40 ice cubes

1,500 mg milk thistle

1,500 mg green tea extract

1. Push the melon, oranges, limes, grapefruits, lemons, mangoes, and blueberries through the juicer. Stir the juice well.

2. Blend the ice cubes, milk thistle, and green tea extract with juice mixture in a blender.

3. Serve immediately.

*Makes 1 Gallon*

# Purple Power Blend

1 cup grapes with seeds, any color

1 medium beet, cubed

½ head red cabbage, chopped

1 cup blueberries

300 mg alpha-lipoic acid

2,000 mg vitamin C

1. Push the grapes, beet, cabbage, and blueberries through the juicer.

2. Stir in the alpha-lipoic acid and vitamin C.

3. Serve immediately.

*Makes 3–4 Cups*

# The Spice of Life

1 watermelon, rind removed, seeded and cubed

1 medium papaya, peeled, pitted, and cubed

1 medium kiwi, peeled and quartered

1 medium pear, cored and quartered

1 cup grapes with seeds, any color

½ bunch spinach, chopped

1 cup chopped collard greens

1 medium zucchini, sliced lengthwise

4 ounces aloe vera juice

½ teaspoon cinnamon

½ teaspoon turmeric

1. Push the fruits and vegetables through the juicer.

2. Blend the aloe vera juice, cinnamon, and turmeric with the juice mixture in a blender.

3. Serve immediately.

*Makes 3–3½ Cups*

# Cardiovascular Health

## Artery Aid

¼ cup pitted cherries

3 medium limes, peeled and quartered

1 cup purple grapes with seeds

3 celery stalks

1 carrot, peeled, sliced lengthwise, top removed

100 mcg vitamin K

200 mg bilberry extract

1. Push all the fruits and vegetables through the juicer. Stir juice well.

2. Stir in the vitamin K and bilberry extract.

3. Serve immediately.

*Makes 2 Cups*

# Cardio Concoction

1 apple, cored and quartered

1 cup chopped spinach

1 cup chopped kale

½ cup chopped chard

½ papaya, peeled, pitted, and cubed

2 cloves garlic, peeled

½-inch piece ginger root

2 tablespoons protein powder

100 mg quercetin

250 mg coenzyme Q10

1.  Push the apple, spinach, kale, chard, papaya, garlic, and ginger through the juicer.

2.  Blend the protein powder, quercetin, and coenzyme Q10 with the juice mixture in a blender.

3.  Serve immediately.

*Makes 2 Cups*

# Smart Heart

½-inch piece ginger root

1 large cucumber, sliced lengthwise

2 celery stalks

2 teaspoons green vegetable powder

1 ounce wakame sea vegetable

1 ounce kombu sea vegetable

1 ounce dulse sea vegetable

150 mg hawthorn berry

1. Push the ginger, cucumber, and celery through the juicer.

2. Blend the green vegetable powder, sea vegetables, and hawthorn berry with the juice mixture in a blender.

3. Serve immediately.

*Makes 1–1½ Cups*

# Strong of Heart

½ small lemon, peeled and quartered

1 small piece organic burdock root

¾ cup dandelion roots

2 cups chopped spinach

1 large pear, cored and quartered

2 apples, cored and quartered

2 ounces aloe vera concentrate

500 mg magnesium

1. Push the lemon, burdock, dandelion, spinach, pear, and apples through the juicer.

2. Add the aloe vera concentrate and magnesium to the juice mixture and stir well.

3. Serve immediately.

*Makes 3 Cups*


# Vitality Shake

½ cup blueberries

1 pear, cored and quartered

1 banana, peeled

4 tablespoons almond butter

½ cup soy milk

1 teaspoon lecithin

100 mg coenzyme Q10

1,500 mg vitamin C

1. Blend all the ingredients in a blender until smooth.

2. Serve immediately.

*Makes 1¼ Cups*

# Cholesterol Health

## Cholesterol Regulator

1 watermelon, rind removed, seeded and cubed

½ pineapple, rind removed, cored and cubed

¼-inch piece ginger root

½ cup seltzer

350 mg black tea extract

¾ cup ice

1. Push the watermelon, pineapple, and ginger through the juicer.

2. Blend the seltzer, black tea extract, and ice with the juice in a blender.

3. Serve chilled.

*Makes 4 Cups*

# Lipoprotein Liquid

½ clove garlic, peeled

2 apples, cored and quartered

2 cups chopped cabbage

1 cup pumpkin, rind removed, seeded and cubed

¼ teaspoon cayenne pepper (optional)

2.5 g apple pectin fiber powder

1. Push the garlic, apples, and cabbage through the juicer.

2. In a food processor, grind the pumpkin.

3. Blend the pumpkin, cayenne, if desired, and apple pectin with the juice mixture in a blender.

4. Serve immediately.

*Makes 2–2½ Cups*

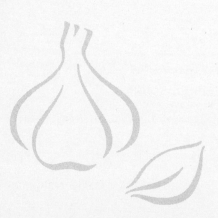

# Cold and Flu

## Flu-Be-Gone

8 ounces soy yogurt

½ teaspoon fructooligosaccharides

2 peeled bananas, frozen

2 cups strawberries, hulled

½ teaspoon powdered probiotic

3 tablespoons raw honey

2,000 mg vitamin C

200 mg beta carotene

1. Blend all the ingredients in a blender or food processor until smooth.

2. Serve immediately.

*Makes 2–3 Cups*


## Fruitful Remedy

1 cup strawberries, hulled and halved

4 carrots, peeled, sliced lengthwise, tops removed

¼ pineapple, rind removed, cored and cubed

500 mg black elderberry extract

125 mg grapefruit seed extract

1. Push the strawberries, carrots, and pineapple through the juicer in the order listed. Stir the juice well.

2. Stir in the black elderberry extract and grapefruit seed extract.

3. Serve immediately.

*Makes 1–2 Cups*

# Immaculate Immunity

¼ small watermelon with rind, cubed

2 cups fresh pitted cherries, prefrozen for 2 or more
hours

2 cups alfalfa sprouts

1 cup blueberries

1 cup raspberries

1 medium peach, pitted and quartered

300 mg green tea extract

1. Push the watermelon, cherries, alfalfa sprouts, blueberries, raspberries, and peach through the juicer. Stir the juice well.

2. Stir in the green tea extract.

3. Serve immediately.

*Makes 2½–3 Cups*

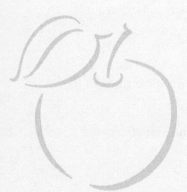

# Rejuvenation Libation

4 large limes, peeled and quartered

1 pineapple, rind removed, cored and quartered

8 large peaches, peeled, pitted, and quartered
   (about 2 cups)

1 small cantaloupe, rind removed, seeded and cubed
   (about 2 cups)

4 peeled bananas, frozen

500 mg alpha-lipoic acid

600 mg curcumin

12 ice cubes

1. Push the limes and pineapple through the juicer.

2. Blend the peaches, cantaloupe, bananas, alpha-lipoic acid, curcumin, and ice cubes with the juice mixture in a blender on high speed until smooth.

3. Serve immediately.

*Makes 12 Cups*

# Sniffle Buster

6–7 carrots, peeled, sliced lengthwise, tops removed

6–7 celery stalks

1 large beet, quartered

1 lemon, peeled and quartered

3 garlic cloves, peeled

1-inch piece ginger root

2 tablespoons raw honey

500 mg goldenseal

250 mg echinacea extract

1. Push the carrots, celery, beet, lemon, garlic, and ginger through the juicer.

2. Add the honey, goldenseal, and echinacea to the juice mixture and stir well.

3. Serve immediately.

*Makes 3 Cups*

# Wintertime Pick-Me-Up

½ medium garlic clove, peeled

¾ cup peeled and quartered red onion

1½ cups black or green olives, pitted

4 medium tangerines, peeled and quartered

3 apples, cored and quartered

2 tablespoons eucalyptus honey

800 mg reishi powder

1. Push the garlic, onion, olives, tangerines, and apples through the juicer.

2. Blend the eucalyptus honey and reishi powder with the juice mixture in a blender.

3. Serve immediately.

*Makes 2–2½ Cups*

# Dental Health

## Healthy Smile

2 cups chopped kale

2 cups chopped parsley

1 cup chopped spinach

1 cup chopped broccoli

½ head cauliflower, chopped

6 celery stalks

1 medium apple, cored and quartered

10,000 IU vitamin A

500 mcg chromium picolinate

1. Push all the vegetables and the apple through the juicer. Stir the juice well.

2. Stir in the vitamin A and chromium picolinate.

3. Serve immediately.

*Makes 3–3½ Cups*

# Terrific Teeth

1 cup chopped spinach

½ cup chopped parsley

2 medium celery stalks

1 medium pineapple, rind removed, cored, and cubed

2 apples, cored and quartered

150 mg coenzyme Q10

1 tablespoon lecithin granules

1. Push all the vegetables and fruits through the juicer.

2. Add the coenzyme Q10 and lecithin granules to the juice mixture and stir well.

3. Serve immediately.

*Makes 3½ Cups*

# Depression

## Mango Mood Enhancer

¼ cup freshly squeezed lemon juice

1 cup vanilla-flavored rice milk

2 large mangoes, peeled, pitted, and cut into 1-inch
cubes

1 eight-ounce container lemon-flavored nondairy yogurt

400 mg magnesium

120 mg ginkgo biloba

16–20 ice cubes

1. Blend all the ingredients in a blender on high speed until smooth and creamy.

2. Serve immediately.

*Makes 3–3½ Cups*

# Strawberry Mint Cooler

8 cups mineral water

4 peppermint tea bags

3 tablespoons honey

6 cups hulled strawberries

2 large limes, peeled and quartered

1,000 mg tyrosine

3,000 mg vitamin C

40 ice cubes

1. In a small saucepan, combine the mineral water and tea bags over moderate heat and simmer, covered, for 8–10 minutes, or until fully brewed. Stir in the honey until well combined and set aside to cool completely.

2. Push the strawberries and limes through the juicer.

3. In a large pitcher, combine the juice mixture, tea, tyrosine, vitamin C, and ice. Stir together until well combined.

4. Serve immediately.

*Makes 11–12 Cups*

# Sunny Elixir

4 cups medium strawberries, hulled

1 medium slice cantaloupe, rind removed

1 cup dandelion flowers and stems

2 ounces wheatgrass juice

2 tablespoons flaxseed oil

1 tablespoon lecithin

1. Push the fruits and vegetables through the juicer.

2. Add the wheatgrass juice, flaxseed oil, and lecithin to the juice mixture and stir well.

3. Serve immediately.

*Makes 3–3½ Cups*

# Vitalize and Energize

4 apples, cored and quartered

2 yams, cubed

1 cup alfalfa sprouts

300 mg Saint-John's-wort extract

One standard serving vitamin B complex (containing at
least 800 mg folic acid)

1. Push the apples, yams, and alfalfa sprouts through the juicer.

2. Stir in the Saint-John's-wort extract and vitamin B complex.

3. Serve immediately.

*Makes 4 Cups*

# Detoxification

## The Big Cleanse

½ clove garlic, peeled

2 cups chopped collard greens

2 cups chopped cauliflower

½ cup cubed red beets

1 cup chopped Swiss chard

2 large apples, cored and quartered

2 ounces wheatgrass juice

1 g dandelion root

3 g chlorella

1.  Push the garlic, collard greens, cauliflower, beets, chard, and apples through the juicer.

2.  Add the wheatgrass juice, dandelion root, and chlorella to the juice mixture and stir well.

3.  Serve immediately.

*Makes 1½–2 Cups*

# Citrus Kick Start

1 medium lemon, peeled and quartered

1 medium lime, peeled and quartered

1 medium cucumber, sliced lengthwise

3 celery stalks

½ teaspoon cayenne pepper

400 mg astragalus

1. Push the lemon, lime, cucumber, and celery through the juicer.

2. Add the cayenne and astragalus to the juice mixture and stir well.

3. Serve immediately.

*Makes 2 Cups*

# The Diuretic Detox

¼ watermelon, rind removed, cubed

½ lemon, peeled and quartered

2 tablespoons green powder supplement (containing spirulina and chlorella)

1. Push the fruits through the juicer. Stir the juice well.

2. Add the green powder to the juice mixture and stir well.

3. Serve immediately.

*Makes 3 Cups*

# Green Detox

2 apples, cored and quartered

3 cups chopped cabbage, any color

1 cup chopped kale

1 cup chopped spinach

1 ounce aloe vera concentrate

3 tablespoons olive oil

250 mg schisandra extract

1. Push the fruit and vegetables through the juicer.

2. Blend the aloe vera concentrate, olive oil, and schisandra extract with the juice mixture in a blender.

3. Serve immediately.

*Makes 3 Cups*

# Purifying Punch

1 medium guava, peeled, seeded, and quartered

3 blood oranges, peeled and quartered

2 small artichokes, halved

1 cup chopped broccoli

1 medium red bell pepper, cored, seeded, and quartered

3 cups chopped celery

milk thistle tincture (drops equivalent to 500 mg 80%
   standarized extract)

1. Push the fruits and vegetables through the juicer.

2. Add the milk thistle tincture to the juice mixture and stir well.

3. Serve immediately.

*Makes 3½–4 Cups*

# Diabetes

## Blood Sugar Balancer

    1 ounce wakame sea vegetable

    1 ounce kombu sea vegetable

    1 ounce dulse sea vegetable

    2 cups chopped arugula

    2 cups chopped red leaf lettuce

    2 cups chopped romaine

    2 apples, cored and quartered

    120 mg ginkgo biloba extract

    500 mg bitter melon

1. Cut the sea vegetables into small pieces and chop in a blender or food processor until very fine.

2. Push the lettuce and apples through the juicer.

3. Add the sea vegetables, ginkgo biloba, and bitter melon to the juice mixture and stir well.

4. Serve immediately.

*Makes 1½–2 Cups*

# Chlorophyll Ya Up

2 cups alfalfa sprouts

2 cups chopped spinach

2 cups chopped collard greens without stems

5 medium asparagus stalks

1 apple, cored and quartered

200 mg bilberry extract

2 tablespoons fiber powder

1. Push all vegetables and apple through the juicer.

2. Add the bilberry extract and fiber powder to the juice mixture and stir well.

3. Serve immediately.

*Makes 4 Cups*

# Gary's Glucose Fix

1 medium artichoke heart

1½ cups chopped cabbage, any color

1 cup green beans, trimmed

3 celery stalks

2 large cucumbers, sliced lengthwise

1,000 mg evening primrose oil

7.5 mg vanadyl sulfate (with 1.5 mg vanadium)

1. Push all the vegetables through the juicer and stir well.

2. Stir in the evening primrose oil and vanadyl sulfate.

3. Serve immediately.

*Makes 3½ Cups*


# Insulin Stabilizer

1 cup grapes with seeds, any color

¼ medium cantaloupe, cubed, rind removed

½ cup chopped broccoli

1 cup chopped collard greens (ends cut off)

1 cup chopped spinach (ends cut off)

3 oranges, peeled and quartered

400 mcg chromium picolinate

250 mg alpha-lipoic acid

1. Push the grapes, cantaloupe, broccoli, collard greens, spinach, and oranges through the juicer. Stir the juice well.

2. Stir in the chromium picolinate and alpha-lipoic acid.

3. Serve immediately.

*Makes 4 Cups*

# Digestive Health

## Alkaline Refreshment

1 cup chopped fresh peppermint leaf

5 celery stalks

3 cucumbers, sliced lengthwise

1 teaspoon triphala powder

probiotic powder (at least 5 billion CFU)

1. Push the peppermint, celery, and cucumbers through the juicer.

2. Stir in the triphala powder and probiotic powder.

3. Serve immediately.

*Makes 2 Cups*

# Clean Colon

½ cup blueberries

½ large pear, cored and quartered

½ medium potato, quartered

3 large apples, cored and quartered

2 tablespoons flaxseeds

2 teaspoons psyllium powder

2 ounces aloe vera juice

3 tablespoons raw honey

1. Push the blueberries, pear, potato, and apples through the juicer.

2. Using a grinder, grind the flaxseeds to a very fine powder.

3. In a blender, on the "whip" setting, blend the flaxseeds, psyllium powder, aloe vera concentrate, and honey with the juice mixture.

4. Serve immediately.

*Makes 3–4 Cups*

# Enzyme Enhancer

1 medium papaya, peeled, pitted, and cubed

¼ large pineapple, rind removed, cored and cubed

6–10 large strawberries, hulled and halved

¼ medium head cabbage, chopped

1 small kiwi, peeled and quartered

½ teaspoon probiotic powder

1.  Push all the ingredients except the probiotic powder through the juicer. Stir the juice well.

2.  Stir in the probiotic powder.

3.  Serve immediately.

*Makes 3–4 Cups*


# Enzyme Express

1-inch piece ginger root

½ cup basil

3 celery stalks

½ head cabbage, any color, chopped

2 medium bananas, peeled

one standard serving digestive enzyme supplement

1.  Push the ginger, basil, celery, and cabbage through the juicer.

2.  Blend the bananas and digestive enzymes with the juice mixture in a blender until smooth.

3.  Serve immediately.

*Makes 3¼ Cups*

# Friendly Fiber Colon Cleanse

¼ cup oat bran

¼ cup hulled buckwheat

¼ cup amaranth

¼ cup millet

3 apples, cored and quartered

½ yam, quartered

2 bananas, peeled

3 tablespoons raw honey

⅛ teaspoon ground cinnamon

1 teaspoon chia seeds

1.  Separately cook the oat bran, buckwheat, amaranth, and millet until soft.

2.  Push the apples and yam through the juicer.

3.  Blend the grains, bananas, honey, cinnamon, and chia seeds with the juice mixture in a blender until smooth.

4.  Serve immediately.

*Makes 3–3½ Cups*


# Good-bye UTI

1 tablespoon flaxseeds

1 papaya, peeled, pitted, and cubed

2 cups cranberries

2 tablespoons fiber powder

1 tablespoon aloe vera concentrate

2,000 mg vitamin C

1.  In a grinder, grind the flaxseeds into a very fine powder.

2. Blend the flaxseeds with remaining ingredients in a blender until smooth.

3. Serve immediately.

*Makes 1½–2 Cups*

# Stomach Settler

6 celery stalks

1-inch piece ginger root

12 mint julep leaves with stems

½ cup blueberries

1 medium apple, cored and quartered

2 ounces aloe vera concentrate

one standard serving digestive enzyme supplement

4 ounces sparkling mineral water

1. Use the celery stalks to push the ginger and mint leaves through the juicer, juicing the celery in the process. Set aside the juice.

2. Push the blueberries and apple through the juicer.

3. Combine the juices and stir well.

4. Add the aloe vera concentrate and digestive enzyme supplement to the juice mixture and stir well.

5. Add the sparkling mineral water to the juice mixture and stir well.

6. Serve immediately.

*Makes 2–2½ Cups*

# Stomach Soother

8 cups mineral water

4 peppermint tea bags

4 ounces fresh ginger root, cut into ½-inch pieces

1½ tablespoons raw honey (optional)

¼ cup freshly squeezed lemon juice

40 ice cubes

1. In a small saucepan, combine the mineral water, tea bags, and ginger over moderate heat and simmer, covered, for 8–10 minutes, or until fully brewed. Sir in the honey, if desired, until well combined and set aside to cool completely.

2. In a large pitcher, combine the tea, lemon juice, and ice. Stir together until well combined.

3. Serve immediately.

*Makes 10 Cups*

# Energy and Stamina

## Endura Max

1 papaya, peeled, pitted, and quartered

1 orange, peeled and quartered

¼ pineapple, rind removed, cored and quartered

2 tablespoons protein powder

400 mg astragalus

1. Push the papaya, orange, and pineapple through the juicer.

2. Add the protein powder and astragalus to the juice mixture and stir well.

3. Serve immediately.

*Makes 1–1½ Cups*

# Fatigue Buster

3 carrots, peeled, sliced lengthwise, tops removed

2 cucumbers, sliced

1 pear, cored and quartered

¼ teaspoon bee propolis

¼ teaspoon guarana powder

1. Push the carrots, cucumbers, and pear through the juicer.

2. Add the bee propolis and guarana to the juice mixture and stir well.

3. Serve immediately.

*Makes 1–1½ Cups*

# Mitochondrial Might

16 large apples, cored and quartered

4 large limes, peeled and quartered

8 large peaches, peeled, pitted, and quartered (about 2 cups)

4 kiwis, peeled and quartered

2 peeled bananas, frozen

1 cup seedless grapes, any color

ground cinnamon to taste

300 mg coenzyme Q10

16–20 ice cubes

1. Push the apples and limes through the juicer.

2. Blend the peaches, kiwis, bananas, grapes, cinnamon, coenzyme Q10, and ice with the juice mixture in a blender on high speed until smooth and creamy.

3. Serve immediately.

*Makes 12 Cups*

# Victory Mix

½ cup nondairy ice cream

½ cup blueberries

½ cup bananas, peeled and sliced

2 tablespoons vegetarian protein powder

6 ounces rice milk or soy milk

250 mg Siberian ginseng

1. Blend all the ingredients together in a blender until smooth.

2. Serve immediately.

*Makes 2–2½ Cups*


# Wherewithal Wonder

1½ cups strawberries, hulled

2 ounces any healthy nutrition bar

4 ounces vanilla soy frozen dessert

2 peeled bananas, frozen

1 cup blueberries

2 ounces whole blueberry soy yogurt

2 tablespoons protein powder

900 mg gotu kola

1. Blend all the ingredients together in a blender or food processor until smooth.

2. Serve immediately.

*Makes 3 Cups*

# Eye Health

## Buena Vista

  2 cups purple grapes with seeds

  2 cups green grapes with seeds

  2 cups chopped spinach

  2 cups chopped kale

  4 ounces mineral water

  5 mg astaxanthin

  150 mg bilberry extract

1.  Push the grapes, spinach, and kale through the juicer.

2.  Add the mineral water, astaxanthin, and bilberry extract to the juice mixture and stir well.

3.  Serve immediately.

*Makes 1½–2 Cups*


## Expanded Vision

  4 cups blueberries

  1 cup coconut milk

  1 tablespoon flaxseed oil

  6 mg lutein

1.  Blend all the ingredients together in a blender until smooth and creamy.

2.  Serve immediately.

*Makes 2 Cups*

# Eye Essentials

1 cup grapes with seeds, any color

1 medium apricot, pitted and halved

1 cup frozen or room-temperature huckleberries

2 cups blueberries

1 cantaloupe, rind removed, cubed

2 medium yams, quartered

1 cup chopped spinach

200 mcg selenium

1,000 IU vitamin E

1. Push the fruits and vegetables through the juicer. Stir the juice well.

2. Stir in the selenium and vitamin E.

3. Serve immediately.

*Makes 4–5 Cups*

# Hair Health

## Follicle Fixer

1 watermelon, rind removed, cut into 1-inch cubes

1 large pineapple, rind removed, cored and cut into
  1-inch cubes

8 large limes, peeled and quartered

120 mg stinging nettle extract

two standard servings vitamin B complex

20–24 ice cubes

1. Push the watermelon, pineapple, and limes through the juicer. Stir the juice well.

2. Stir in the stinging nettle extract and vitamin B complex.

3. Serve immediately.

*Makes 1 Gallon*

# Hair Repair Juice

8 cups mineral water

4 decaffeinated green tea bags

¼ cup honey (optional)

2 pineapples, rind removed, cored and cubed

16 kiwis, peeled and quartered, plus kiwi slices for
    garnish (optional)

4 large limes, peeled and quartered

2 tablespoons coconut oil

40 ice cubes

fresh mint to taste

1. In a small saucepan, combine the mineral water and tea bags over moderate heat and simmer, covered, for 8–10 minutes, or until fully brewed. Sir in the honey, if desired, until well combined and set aside to cool completely.

2. Push the pineapples, kiwis, and limes through the juicer.

3. In a large pitcher, combine the juice mixture, tea, coconut oil, and ice. Stir together until well combined.

4. Pour into glasses and garnish with kiwi slices, if desired, and mint.

5. Serve immediately.

*Makes 1½ Gallons*

# Healthy Roots

3 burdock roots, peeled and sliced

2 parsnips, sliced

4 carrots, peeled, sliced lengthwise, tops removed

1 cup chopped parsley greens

1 tablespoon blackstrap molasses

500 mg evening primrose oil

1,000 mg vitamin C

1. Push the burdock, parsnips, carrots, and parsley greens through the juicer.

2. Blend the molasses, evening primrose oil, and vitamin C with the juice mixture in a blender.

3. Serve immediately.

*Makes 2 Cups*

# Headaches

## Pain-Free Potion

16 oranges, peeled and quartered

8 limes, peeled and quartered

2 cups mixed berries (strawberries, raspberries,
blackberries, and boysenberries), hulled

450 mg feverfew

400 mg magnesium

1. Push the oranges, limes, and berries through the juicer.

2. Stir in the feverfew and magnesium.

3. Serve immediately.

*Makes 7 Cups*

## Tension Relief

3 tablespoons flaxseeds

1 cup puffed rice

1 cup tofu yogurt

½ cup plain rice milk

one standard serving vitamin B complex

125 mg ginkgo biloba

1. In a grinder, grind the flaxseeds into a very fine powder.

2. In a blender, chop the puffed rice.

3. Add the flaxseeds and remaining ingredients to blender and
blend until smooth.

4. Serve chilled.

*Makes 1–1½ Cups*

# Insomnia

## Renewing Rest

2 ripe papayas, peeled, pitted, and quartered

½ apple, cored and quartered

1 cup chopped spinach

valerian root extract (equivalent to 500 mg of
   dried herb)

1.  Push the papayas, apple, and spinach through the juicer.
    Stir the juice well.

2.  Stir in the valerian root extract.

3.  Serve immediately.

*Makes 1–1½ Cups*

## Sleepy Elixir

4 sweet potatoes, peeled and cut into 2-inch cubes

4 cups vanilla-flavored rice milk

4 peeled bananas, frozen

1 tablespoon pure vanilla extract

ground cinnamon to taste

ground nutmeg to taste

500 mg passionflower

400 mg skullcap

16–20 ice cubes

1.  To cook the sweet potatoes, place the potato pieces on a
    steamer set into a large pot filled with 1 inch of mineral
    water. Cook, covered, over high heat for 10–15 minutes, or

until the potato pieces are tender when a fork is inserted into their centers. Remove the steamer and run the potatoes under cold water until they are cool.

2. Blend the potatoes, rice milk, bananas, vanilla extract, cinnamon, nutmeg, passionflower, and skullcap in a blender on high speed until smooth and creamy.

3. Pour into tall glasses filled with ice and serve immediately.

*Makes 11 Cups*

# Tea Time Relaxer

    1 chamomile tea bag
    1 cup mineral water, boiled
    1 papaya, peeled, pitted, and cubed
    1 mango, peeled, pitted, and cubed
    1 banana, peeled and sliced
    5 mg melatonin

1. Steep the chamomile tea in 1 cup hot mineral water for 15 minutes and allow the tea to cool completely.

2. Blend the tea with the papaya, mango, banana, and melatonin in a blender until smooth.

3. Serve immediately.

*Makes 3 Cups*

# Liver Health

## Liver Cleanse

    1 cup chopped chard

    1 cup chopped spinach

    3 apples, cored and quartered

    1 avocado, peeled, pitted, and cubed

    1 tablespoon finely diced peppermint leaves (or
        peppermint oil, to taste, if desired)

    ⅛ teaspoon cayenne pepper

    milk thistle tincture (drops equivalent to 500 mg
        80% standarized extract)

1. Push the chard, spinach, and apples through the juicer.

2. Blend the avocado, peppermint, cayenne, and milk thistle with the juice mixture until smooth. (If preferred, peppermint oil, to taste, may be substituted for the diced peppermint leaves.)

3. Serve immediately.

*Makes 1½ Cups*

## Liver and Gall Flush

    1 cup Brussels sprouts

    4 large cucumbers, sliced lengthwise

    2 cups chopped cabbage, any color

    1½ cups cauliflower

    2 medium apples, cored and quartered

    1 medium avocado, pitted

1 g dandelion root

125 mg inositol

1.  Push the Brussels sprouts, cucumbers, cabbage, cauliflower, and apples through the juicer.

2.  Blend the avocado, dandelion root, and inositol with the juice mixture in a blender until smooth.

3.  Serve immediately.

*Makes 4–5 Cups*

# Lupus

## Invigorating Blend

3 tablespoons flaxseeds

1 carrot, peeled, sliced lengthwise, top removed

½ cup cantaloupe, cubed, rind removed

1 cup mineral water

25 mg DHEA

1.  In a grinder, grind the flaxseeds into a very fine powder.

2.  Push the carrot and cantaloupe through the juicer.

3.  Combine the flaxseed powder, juice mixture, mineral water, and DHEA and stir well. (Diluted juice is easier to digest.)

4.  Keep refrigerated and serve over the course of 1–2 days.

*Makes 1½ Cups*

# Muscle Support Mix

1 carrot, peeled, sliced lengthwise, top removed

¼ cup chopped dates

1 cup soy milk

3 peeled bananas, frozen

2 tablespoons rice protein powder

1. Push all the ingredients except the rice protein powder through the juicer.

2. Stir in the rice protein powder.

3. Serve immediately.

*Makes 2–2¼ Cups*


# Tissue Tonic

1 papaya, peeled, pitted, and cubed

1 cup cranberries

2 oranges, peeled and quartered

1 cup coconut milk

500 mg cat's claw

1. Push the papaya, cranberries, and oranges through the juicer.

2. Blend the coconut milk and cat's claw with the juice mixture in a blender.

3. Serve immediately.

*Makes 3–4 Cups*

# Menopause

## Balancing Brew

2 medium whole cucumbers, sliced

1 medium apple, cored and quartered

½ medium lemon, peeled and quartered

¾ cup grapes with seeds, any color

1 cup cubed watermelon, rind removed

one standard serving of vitamin B complex

black cohosh root extract (drops equivalent to 250 mg of
dried herb)

1. Push the cucumbers and fruits through the juicer.

2. Stir in the vitamin B complex and black cohosh root extract.

3. Serve immediately.

*Makes 2½–3 Cups*

# Equilibrium Elixir

2 cups raspberries

1 large ripe peach, peeled, pitted, and quartered

2 peeled bananas, frozen

2 tablespoons soy protein powder

½ cup plain soy yogurt

4 ounces soy milk

1,000 mg vitamin C

1. Push the raspberries and peach through the juicer.

2. Blend the bananas, soy protein powder, yogurt, soy milk, and vitamin C with the juice mixture until smooth.

3. Serve immediately.

*Makes 3 Cups*


# Healthy Woman

2 green bell peppers, cored, seeded, and quartered

2 apples, cored and quartered

200 mg wild yam

400 mg dong quai

1. Push the bell peppers and apples through the juicer. Stir the juice well.

2. Stir in the wild yam and dong quai.

3. Serve immediately.

*Makes 1–1½ Cups*

# Muscle Building

## Decathlon Smoothie

2 teaspoons rice protein powder

1 tablespoon soy protein powder

1 banana, peeled

10 ounces bottled apple juice

2,000 mg vitamin C

3 g L-glutamine

1. Blend all the ingredients together in a blender until smooth.
2. Serve immediately.

*Makes 1½–2 Cups*


## Gary's Muscle Shake

2 heaping tablespoons protein powder with branched
   chain amino acids

1 banana, peeled

8 ounces bottled apple juice

1 g creatine supplement

¼ teaspoon allspice

1. Blend all the ingredients together in a blender until smooth.
2. Serve immediately.

*Makes 2 Cups*

# Muscle Performance

1 large pear, cored and quartered

½ large apple, peeled, cored, and quartered

1 peeled banana, frozen

3 scoops vegetarian protein powder with branched chain
   amino acids

7 tablespoons creamy peanut butter

½ cup vanilla soy ice cream

200 mg Korean ginseng

10–12 ice cubes

1.  Push the pear and apple through the juicer.

2.  Separately, blend the banana, protein powder, peanut butter, soy ice cream, ginseng, and ice cubes in a blender or food processor until smooth.

3.  Add the juice to the blended mixture and blend until well combined.

4.  Serve immediately.

*Makes 3–4 Cups*

# Nature's Finest Protein Shake

2½ cups vanilla soy milk

2 cups blueberries

2 peeled bananas, frozen

3 tablespoons soy butter

3 tablespoons almond butter

3 tablespoons cashew butter

3 tablespoons macadamia butter

3 tablespoons sunflower butter

1. Blend the soy milk, blueberries, and bananas in a blender or food processor.

2. Add the butters to the blended mixture and blend until smooth.

3. Serve immediately.

*Makes 3½–4 Cups*

# Workout Special

2 scoops vegetarian protein powder

2 tablespoons almond butter

2 ounces vanilla soy milk

2 ounces soft tofu

2 tablespoons raw maca powder

1 medium tomato, quartered

1 yam, quartered

4 medium celery stalks

5 ice cubes

1. Blend the protein powder, almond butter, soy milk, tofu, and maca powder in a blender until smooth.

2. Push the tomato, yam, and celery through the juicer.

3. Combine the juice mixture and blended mixture in a shaker with ice and shake until frothy.

4. Serve immediately.

*Makes 2–2½ Cups*

# Osteoporosis

## Bone Health Smoothie

½ honeydew melon, rind removed, cubed

1 banana, peeled

¼ cup agar-agar

½ cup soy milk

1,000 IU vitamin $D_3$

200 mg calcium citrate

1. Push the honeydew through the juicer.

2. Blend the banana, agar-agar, and soy milk with the juice of the honeydew in a blender until smooth.

3. Stir in the vitamin D and calcium citrate.

4. Serve immediately.

*Makes 2 Cups*

# Bone Mass Booster

1 cup sliced asparagus

1 cup sliced cucumbers

2 ounces chopped parsley

½ cup pitted black olives

½ apple, cored and quartered

2 medium carrots, peeled, sliced lengthwise, tops
   removed

2 ounces coconut milk

100 mg dried plum extract

200 mg magnesium

1. Push the asparagus, cucumbers, parsley, olives, apple, and carrots through the juicer.

2. Add the coconut milk, dried plum extract, and magnesium to the juice mixture and stir well.

3. Serve immediately.

*Makes 2–3 Cups*


# Joint Aid

3 large cucumbers, sliced lengthwise

½ cup blueberries

1 apple, cored and quartered

50 mg DHEA

½ teaspoon flaxseed oil

1. Push the cucumbers, blueberries, and apple through the juicer. Stir the juice well.

2. Stir in the DHEA and flaxseed oil.

3. Serve immediately.

*Makes 1½ Cups*

# Premenstrual Syndrome (PMS)

## Beat the Heat

1 large bunch flat-leaf parsley (about ¼ pound)

8 large tomatoes, quartered

8 large celery stalks

4 large carrots, peeled, sliced lengthwise, tops removed

4 yellow bell peppers, cored, seeded, and quartered

4 large limes, peeled

sea salt to taste (about ½ teaspoon)

1,000 mg magnesium

chasteberry extract (drops equivalent to 800 mg dried
herb)

1. Bunch up the parsley and push through the juicer.

2. Juice tomatoes, celery, carrots, bell peppers, and limes.

3. Add the salt, magnesium, and chasteberry extract to the juice
mixture and stir well.

4. Serve immediately.

*Makes 12 Cups*

# Feminine Fix

1 medium cucumber, quartered lengthwise

5 medium celery stalks

1 medium tomato, quartered

1 teaspoon kelp powder

1,000 mg evening primrose oil

1. Push the cucumber, celery, and tomato through the juicer.

2. Add the kelp powder and evening primrose oil to the juice mixture and stir well.

3. Serve immediately.

*Makes 2–2½ Cups*


# Minty Relief

¼ cup mint julep leaves

4 ounces coconut water

2 tablespoons carob powder

4 ounces vanilla-flavored rice milk

3 drops peppermint oil

1 teaspoon brown rice syrup

5 ice cubes

1. Push the mint julep leaves through the juicer.

2. Blend the remaining ingredients with the juice mixture in a blender until smooth.

3. Serve immediately.

*Makes 1–1½ Cups*

# Prostate Health

## Endocrine Enhancement

4 medium carrots, peeled, sliced lengthwise,
  tops removed
½ cup chopped parsley
2 cups chopped spinach
½ medium apple, cored and quartered
2 tablespoons pumpkin seeds
120 mg stinging nettle extract
150 mg saw palmetto extract

1. Use the carrots to push the parsley, spinach, and apple through the juicer, juicing the carrots in the process.

2. Using a food processor, grind the pumpkin seeds into a very fine powder.

3. Add the pumpkin seed powder, stinging nettle extract, and saw palmetto extract to the juice mixture and stir well.

4. Serve immediately.

*Makes 2–2½ Cups*

# Lycopene Supreme

    7 ounces vanilla soy milk
    4 dates, pitted
    150 mg saw palmetto extract
    15 mg lycopene

1.  Blend all the ingredients in a blender until smooth.

2.  Serve chilled.

*Makes 1 Cup*


# Prostate Pro

    3 cucumbers, sliced lengthwise
    1 lime, peeled and halved
    3 kiwis, peeled and quartered
    1 teaspoon blackstrap molasses
    30 mg zinc
    1 g bee pollen

1.  Push the cucumbers, lime, and kiwis through the juicer.

2.  Blend the blackstrap molasses, zinc, and bee pollen with the juice mixture in a blender.

3.  Serve over ice.

*Makes 1–1½ Cups*

# Respiratory Health

## Asthma Relief

    1 medium watermelon with rind, cubed

    8 kiwis, peeled

    2 grapefruits, peeled and quartered

    2 limes, peeled and quartered

    1 lemon, peeled and quartered

    1,000 mg quercetin

    400 mg bromelain

1.  Push the watermelon, kiwis, grapefruits, limes, and lemon through the juicer. Stir the juice well.

2.  Mix in the quercetin and bromelain.

3.  Serve immediately.

*Makes 14 Cups*

# Breathe Easy Brew

1 cup pecan halves

4 cups mineral water for soaking, plus 4 cups
   mineral water

2 tablespoons raw local honey

1 tablespoon pure almond flavor

2 teaspoons pure vanilla extract

pinch of salt

400 mg magnesium

400 mg deglycyrrhizinated licorice root extract
   (10:1 ratio)

1.  Soak the pecan halves in 4 cups mineral water for 6–8 hours, then discard the soaking water and rinse well.

2.  Blend the prepared pecans and 4 cups mineral water in a blender on medium speed for 30 seconds, increase the speed to high, and continue blending for about 1 minute, or until homogenous.

3.  Transfer the blended pecan mixture to a cheesecloth-lined fine sieve and strain into a medium-sized bowl (squeeze or use a spoon to stir and push the pecan milk through while you pour, since it will be too rich to strain it through without a bit of mashing). Save the pulp for hot cereal, grain dishes, baked goods, or smoothies.

4.  Rinse and dry the blender, then pour in the strained pecan milk, honey, almond flavor, vanilla extract, salt, magnesium, and licorice root extract. Blend on high speed until smooth and frothy, about 1 minute.

5.  Transfer to a container and refrigerate for 1–2 hours, or until chilled.

*Makes 4–6 Cups*

# Respiration Libation

2 cups chopped kale

2 cups chopped spinach

2 cloves garlic

2 celery stalks

2 teaspoons green vegetable powder

500 mg cordyceps mushroom powder

1. Push the kale, spinach, garlic, and celery through the juicer.

2. Blend the green vegetable powder and cordyceps mushroom powder with the juice mixture in a blender.

3. Serve immediately.

*Makes 1½–2 Cups*


# Strong Lungs

1 apple, cored and quartered

½ large guava, peeled, seeded, and quartered

6 large carrots, peeled, sliced lengthwise, tops removed

1 avocado, peeled, pitted, and quartered

3 teaspoons liquid chlorophyll

1. Push the fruits and vegetables through the juicer.

2. Add the liquid chlorophyll to the juice mixture and stir well.

3. Serve immediately.

*Makes 4 Cups*

# Skin Health

## Ageless Antidote

1 grapefruit, peeled and cut into small chunks

1 pear, cored and cut into small chunks

¾ cup strawberries, hulled

¾ cup blueberries

1,500 mg vitamin C

½ teaspoon flaxseed oil

½ cup ice

1. Blend all the ingredients together in a blender until smooth.

2. Serve immediately.

*Makes 3 Cups*


## Beauty Shake

7 cucumbers, peeled and sliced lengthwise

1 lemon, peeled and quartered

1 avocado, peeled and pitted

2 tablespoons aloe vera concentrate

one standard serving vitamin B complex (containing
600 mcg biotin)

1. Push the cucumbers and lemon through the juicer.

2. Blend the avocado, aloe vera concentrate, and vitamin B complex with the juice mixture in a blender.

3. Serve immediately.

*Makes 2–3 Cups*

# Complexion Concoction

1 medium cucumber, sliced lengthwise

3 medium parsnips, cubed

3 large carrots, peeled, sliced lengthwise, tops removed

1 large pineapple, rind removed, cored and cubed

10,000 IU vitamin A

2,000 mg vitamin C

1. Push the cucumber, parsnips, carrots, and pineapple through the juicer. Stir the juice well.

2. Stir in the vitamin A and vitamin C.

3. Serve immediately.

*Makes 5 Cups*

# Kiwi Skin Complex

8 cups mineral water

4 decaffeinated green tea bags

¼ cup honey (optional)

2 pineapples, rind removed, cored and cubed

16 kiwis, peeled and quartered

4 large limes, peeled and quartered

2,000 IU vitamin E

20,000 IU vitamin A

40 ice cubes

1. In a small saucepan, combine the mineral water and tea bags over moderate heat and simmer, covered, for 8–10 minutes, or until fully brewed. Sir in the honey, if desired, until well combined and set aside to cool completely.

2. Push the pineapples, kiwis, and limes through the juicer.

3. In a large pitcher, combine the juice mixture, tea, vitamin E, vitamin A, and ice. Stir together until well combined.

4. Serve immediately.

*Makes 1½ Gallons*

# Raw Radiance

½ honeydew melon, cubed, rind removed

2 yams, peeled and quartered

500 mcg chromium picolinate

40 mg zinc

1. Push the honeydew and yams through the juicer and stir juice well.

2. Stir in the chromium picolinate and zinc.

3. Serve immediately.

*Makes 2 Cups*


# Wrinkle Free

1 potato, quartered

2 apples, peeled, cored, quartered

400 mg green tea extract

500 mg burdock root

1. Push the potato and apples through the juicer in the order listed and stir the juice well.

2. Stir in the green tea extract and burdock root.

3. Serve immediately.

*Makes 1–1½ Cups*

# Stress Relief

## Calm Breeze Cooler

2 decaffeinated green tea bags

4 cups mineral water

4 large oranges, peeled and quartered

2 large limes, peeled and quartered

1 large lemon, peeled and quartered

1 cup unsweetened cranberry juice

2 cups blueberries

¼ cup honey

1 teaspoon ground cinnamon

40 ice cubes

400 mg Saint-John's-wort (0.3 percent hypericin content)

1.  In a small saucepan, add the tea bags to the mineral water and simmer over moderate heat, covered, for 8–10 minutes, or until fully brewed. Set aside and allow to cool completely.

2.  Push the oranges, limes, and lemon through the juicer.

3.  Blend the tea, orange juice mixture, cranberry juice, blueberries, honey, cinnamon, half the ice cubes, and Saint-John's-wort in a blender on high speed until well combined.

4.  Pour into glasses filled with the remaining ice cubes.

5.  Serve immediately.

*Makes 8 Cups*

# De-stress Express

5 celery stalks

3 large carrots, peeled, sliced lengthwise, tops removed

½ apple, cored and sliced

ground ginger to taste

200 mg kava kava

100 mg theanine

1. Push the celery, carrots, and apple through the juicer.

2. Add the dash of ginger, the kava kava, and the theanine to the juice mixture and stir well.

3. Serve immediately.

*Makes 1–1½ Cups*


# Peaceful Punch

1 large Golden Delicious apple, cored and quartered

½ cup cranberries

½ cup blueberries

1 cup dandelion roots and leaves

½ cup soy yogurt

200 mg phosphatidyl serine

1. Use the apple to push the cranberries, blueberries, and dandelion roots and leaves through the juicer, juicing the apple in the process.

2. Blend the soy yogurt and phosphatidyl serine with the juice mixture in a blender until smooth.

3. Serve immediately.

*Makes 1½–2 Cups*

# Tranquillity Tonic

4 celery stalks

3 carrots, peeled, sliced lengthwise, tops removed

2 apples, cored and quartered

1-inch piece ginger root

25 mg chamomile leaves

¼ teaspoon nutmeg

¼ teaspoon cinnamon

1. Push the celery, carrots, apples, and ginger through the juicer.

2. Add the chamomile to the juice mixture and stir well.

3. Blend the nutmeg and cinnamon with the juice mixture in a blender.

4. Serve immediately.

*Makes 3 Cups*

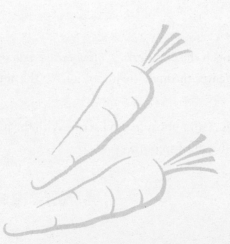

# Weight Loss

## Gary's Get-Up-and-Go Ginger Ale

1-inch piece ginger root

½ large cantaloupe with rind, cubed

1 cup strawberries, hulled and halved

1 medium orange, peeled and quartered

4 ounces sparkling mineral water

400 mg Korean ginseng

1.  Push the ginger, cantaloupe, strawberries, and orange through the juicer.

2.  Add the sparkling mineral water and ginseng to the juice mixture and stir well.

3.  Serve immediately.

*Makes 2 Cups*

## Healthy and Slim

2 apples, cored and quartered

4 celery stalks

2 cucumbers, sliced lengthwise

2 tablespoons protein powder

400 mg green tea extract

⅛ teaspoon cayenne pepper

1.  Push the apples, celery, and cucumbers through the juicer.

2.  Blend the protein powder, green tea extract, and cayenne with the juice mixture in a blender.

3.  Serve immediately.

*Makes 2 Cups*

# Kiss Your Fat Good-bye

2 cups chopped kale

1-inch piece ginger root

6 medium carrots, peeled, sliced lengthwise, tops
   removed

1 cup cubed watermelon, rind removed

1 cup chopped parsley

½ small lemon, peeled and quartered

1 medium artichoke heart, halved

400 mg green coffee extract

1.   Push the kale, ginger, carrots, watermelon, parsley, lemon,
and artichoke heart through the juicer. Stir the juice well.

2.   Stir in the green coffee extract.

3.   Serve immediately.

*Makes 4–5 Cups*

# Lean and Mean Juice

1 large bunch flat-leaf parsley (about ¼ pound)

4 large cucumbers, cut into quarters lengthwise

4 pears, cored and quartered

1-inch piece ginger root

1,000 mg L-carnitine

2 tablespoon lecithin

1. Bunch up the parsley and push it through the juicer.

2. Push cucumbers, pears, and ginger through juicer. Stir the juice well.

3. Stir in the L-carnitine and lecithin.

4. Serve immediately.

*Makes 4 Cups*


# Metabolism Master

2 kiwis, peeled and quartered

2 passion fruits, quartered

3 tangerines, peeled and quartered

1 grapefruit, peeled and quartered

5 celery stalks, leaves removed

½ teaspoon cayenne pepper

150 mg African mango extract

8 ice cubes

1. Push the kiwis, passion fruits, tangerines, grapefruit, and celery through the juicer. Stir the juice well.

2. Stir in the cayenne and African mango extract.

3. Pour over ice and serve immediately.

*Makes 4–5 Cups*

# BREAKFAST FOODS

# A Live Breakfast Porridge

1 cup quinoa

4 cups mineral water

12 large apples, cored and quartered

8 large peaches, peeled, pitted, and sliced (about 4
    cups)

2 cups pitted cherries

ground cinnamon to taste

1. In a medium-sized mixing bowl, combine the quinoa and mineral water. Cover and set aside to soak until the quinoa is just tender, but not soft, 12–24 hours. Discard any excess soaking water, rinse well, drain, and set aside.

2. Push the apples through the juicer.

3. Spoon quinoa into bowls and serve warm or chilled, topped with apple juice, peaches, cherries, and cinnamon.

*Makes 5 Servings*

# Hearty Oats with Nuts and Raisins

4 pears, cored and quartered (1 cup juice)

1 cup mineral water

1 cup rolled oats

1 banana, peeled and sliced

¼ cup raisins

¼ cup chopped unsalted black walnuts

½ teaspoon pure vanilla extract

dash of ground cinnamon

1. Push the pears through the juicer. Set aside 1 cup of the juice.

2. In a medium-sized saucepan, combine the mineral water and pear juice and bring to a boil over high heat.

3. Reduce the heat to medium-low and stir in the oats. Cook uncovered for 5 minutes, stirring occasionally.

4. Add the remaining ingredients and cook for an additional 5 minutes, stirring occasionally.

5. Serve hot with unsweetened soy milk.

*Makes 2 Servings*

# Carrot Sunflower Granola

2 carrots, peeled, sliced lengthwise, tops removed
   (½ cup pulp)

1 cup rolled oats

½ cup whole unsalted almonds

¼ cup raisins

¼ cup unsalted hulled sunflower seeds

½ cup pure maple syrup

2 teaspoons pure almond extract

½ teaspoon ground cinnamon

1. Preheat the oven to 375°F.

2. Push the carrots through the juicer and set aside ½ cup of the pulp.

3. In a large mixing bowl, combine the carrot pulp with the remaining ingredients, mixing well.

4. Spread the mixture on a greased 15-by-20-inch cookie sheet and bake for 15 minutes, or until the top of the mixture turns brown.

5. Serve hot over ice cream or cold with unsweetened soy milk.

*Makes 2 Servings*

# Barley Cereal with Apples and Spice

4 oranges, peeled and quartered (1 cup juice)

2 apples, peeled and quartered (½ cup pulp)

½ cup mineral water

⅓ cup pearl barley

⅓ cup whole dried apricots

3 tablespoons pure maple syrup

½ teaspoon ground cinnamon

1. Separately push the oranges and the apples through the juicer. Set aside 1 cup of the orange juice and ½ cup of the apple pulp.

2. In a medium-sized saucepan, combine the orange juice and mineral water and bring to a boil over high heat.

3. Reduce the heat to medium-low and stir in the barley. Cook uncovered for 10–15 minutes, stirring occasionally.

4. Add the apple pulp and the remaining ingredients and cook for an additional 5–10 minutes, stirring occasionally.

5. Serve hot with unsweetened soy milk or juice.

*Makes 2 Servings*

# Sweet Rice Cream Cereal

4 apples, cored and quartered (1 cup juice and 2
　　tablespoons pulp)
½–¾ cup mineral water
1½ cups unsweetened soy milk
½ cup short-grain brown rice
¼ cup raisins
¼ cup unsalted chopped pecans
2 tablespoons light-colored honey (clover, tupelo, or
　　wildflower)
½ teaspoon pure vanilla extract
¼ teaspoon ground cinnamon

1. Push the apples through the juicer. Set aside 1 cup of the juice and 2 tablespoons of the pulp.

2. In a large saucepan, combine the apple juice, mineral water, and soy milk, and bring to a boil over high heat.

3. Reduce the heat to low and stir in the rice. Cover and continue cooking until the water is absorbed, about 30 minutes.

4. Add the apple pulp and the remaining ingredients and stir.

5. Serve hot with unsweetened soy milk or juice.

*Makes 2 Servings*

# Cream of Rice with Peaches and Honey

3 peaches, peeled, pitted, and sliced (¾ cup pulp)

1½ cups mineral water

1 cup unsweetened soy milk

⅓ cup cream of brown rice cereal or farina

2 tablespoons light-colored honey (clover, tupelo, or wildflower)

½ cup chopped dates

½ teaspoon pure almond extract

dash of ground nutmeg

1. Push the peaches through the juicer. Set aside ¾ cup of the pulp.

2. In a medium-sized saucepan, combine the mineral water and soy milk and bring to a boil over high heat.

3. Reduce the heat to medium-low and stir in the cream of brown rice or farina. Cook uncovered for 3–4 minutes, stirring occasionally.

4. Add the peach pulp and the remaining ingredients and cook for an additional 3–4 minutes, stirring occasionally.

5. Serve hot with unsweetened soy milk or juice.

*Makes 2 Servings*

# Tropical Millet Delight

6 apples, cored and quartered (1½ cups juice)

1 cup mineral water

½ cup millet

¼ cup mashed banana

2 tablespoons chopped dates

1 tablespoon unsweetened flaked coconut

½ teaspoon pure almond extract

1. Push the apples through the juicer. Set aside 1½ cups of the juice.

2. In a large saucepan, combine the mineral water and apple juice and bring to a boil over high heat.

3. Reduce the heat to medium-low and stir in the millet. Cook uncovered until the water is absorbed, about 10 minutes.

4. Add the remaining ingredients and stir.

5. Serve hot with unsweetened soy milk or juice.

*Makes 2 Servings*

# Cocoa Kasha with Bananas

4 apples, cored and quartered (1 cup juice)

1 cup mineral water

½ cup unsweetened soy milk

⅓ cup kasha

½ cup mashed banana

½ tablespoon pure unsweetened cocoa powder
(unsweetened carob powder may be substituted)

¼ cup pure maple syrup

dash of ground cinnamon

1. Push the apples through the juicer. Set aside 1 cup of the juice.

2. In a medium-sized saucepan, combine the apple juice, mineral water, and soy milk, and bring to a boil over high heat.

3. Reduce the heat to medium-low and stir in the kasha. Cook uncovered for 3–4 minutes, stirring occasionally.

4. Add the remaining ingredients and cook for an additional 3–4 minutes, stirring occasionally.

5. Serve hot with unsweetened soy milk or juice.

*Makes 2 Servings*

# Heavenly Roasted Nuts

1 cup walnuts

1 tablespoon honey

1 teaspoon extra virgin olive oil

1 teaspoon freshly squeezed lemon juice

1.  Preheat oven to 350°F. Line an 11-by-15-inch cookie sheet with parchment paper and set aside.

2.  In a medium-sized mixing bowl, toss together the nuts, honey, oil, and lemon juice until well combined.

3.  Evenly spread the nuts on the prepared sheet. Bake on the middle rack of the preheated oven for 8–10 minutes, or until the nuts are golden. Remove the sheet from the oven and slide the parchment paper to a wire rack until the nuts are completely cool (about 10 minutes).

4.  Serve alone or use these as a topping for cereal, salads, nondairy yogurt, or nondairy frozen dessert.

*Makes About 1 Cup*

# Banana Pecan Pancakes

6 apples, cored and quartered (1½ cups juice)

1 carrot, peeled, sliced lengthwise, top removed
   (¼ cup pulp)

vegetarian egg substitute for 2 eggs

¼ cup pure maple syrup

½ cup mineral water

1 cup whole wheat flour

2 teaspoons baking powder

½ cup toasted wheat germ

½ cup sliced bananas

¼ cup unsalted pecans, halved or chopped

2 tablespoons raisins

½ teaspoon ground cinnamon

2 tablespoons cold-pressed flavorless safflower oil

1. Separately push the apples and the carrot through the juicer. Set aside 1½ cups of the apple juice and ¼ cup of the carrot pulp.

2. In a large mixing bowl, combine the apple juice, egg substitute, maple syrup, and mineral water, mixing well.

3. Stir in the flour, baking powder, and wheat germ, mixing well.

4. Stir in the carrot pulp, bananas, pecans, raisins, and cinnamon.

5. For each pancake, heat 1 tablespoon of oil in a small (6- or 8-inch) frying pan over medium heat. When the oil is hot, pour half the batter into the frying pan so that the bottom of the pan is covered with batter. Let the pancake cook for 2–3 minutes, or until the underside is brown.

6.	Flip the pancake over and reduce the heat to low. Cut the pancake into 8 wedges to allow the center to cook. Cook for an additional 2 minutes, or until the center is done.

7.	Serve hot with unsweetened soy milk or juice.

*Makes 2 Servings*

# Tex-Mex Tofu Scrambler

½ cup sunflower seeds

4 one-ounce slices tempeh bacon

6 tablespoons extra virgin olive oil

¼ cup lecithin granules (optional)

1 teaspoon onion powder

1 teaspoon dry mustard

1 teaspoon dried basil

½ teaspoon ground turmeric

½ teaspoon ground cumin

½ teaspoon celery salt

½ teaspoon sea salt

1 pound soft tofu, well drained and crumbled

1 cup sliced mushrooms

3 tablespoons tamari soy sauce

1 six-ounce Vidalia onion, peeled and finely chopped

4 large cloves garlic, peeled and finely chopped

1 eight-ounce yellow bell pepper, cored, seeded, and
   finely chopped

½ cup finely chopped zucchini

1 six-ounce tomato, finely chopped

1 ripe Hass avocado, peeled, halved, pitted, and finely
   chopped

1 teaspoon balsamic vinegar

½ cup finely chopped fresh cilantro

freshly ground black pepper to taste (optional)

2 large limes, sliced into 1-inch-thick wedges
   (optional)

1. In a large cast-iron frying pan, over moderate to low heat,
   roast the sunflower seeds until golden and transfer to a small
   dish. Set aside.

2.  To broil the tempeh, preheat the broiler and brush the above cast-iron frying pan with 2 tablespoons oil. Evenly space the tempeh in the pan and broil in the preheated oven for about 5 minutes, or until golden. Remove the pan from the oven, transfer the "bacon" to a paper-towel-lined plate, and set aside.

3.  In a small mixing bowl, combine the lecithin, if desired, onion powder, mustard, basil, turmeric, cumin, celery salt, and sea salt. Stir together until well combined and set aside.

4.  In a large mixing bowl, toss together 2 tablespoons of the oil with the tofu and the spice mixture until well combined. Set aside.

5.  In the cast-iron frying pan, combine the remaining 2 tablespoons oil with the mushrooms and tamari. Toss together until well mixed and broil in the preheated oven for about 5 minutes, or until the mushrooms are golden. Remove the pan from the oven and toss in the prepared tofu, onion, garlic, bell pepper, zucchini, tomato, avocado, vinegar, cilantro, and black pepper, if desired, until well combined. Return to the broiler and broil, mixing occasionally, until golden, about 10 minutes.

6.  Serve hot, garnished with "bacon," sunflower seeds, and lime wedges, if desired, and accompanied by whole grain toast.

*Makes 4–6 Servings*

# SOUPS

# Classic Vegetable Stock

1 carrot, peeled, sliced lengthwise, top removed (¼ cup
     juice, plus pulp)

1 celery stalk (¼ cup juice, plus pulp)

3 green bell peppers, cored, seeded, and quartered
     (¼ cup juice, plus pulp)

1¼ cups mineral water

¼ cup chopped yellow onion

1 clove garlic, crushed

1 tablespoon extra virgin olive oil

1 teaspoon chopped fresh thyme, or ½ teaspoon
     dried thyme

½ teaspoon celery seeds

1 bay leaf

1 teaspoon sea salt

½ teaspoon black pepper

1. Separately push the carrot, celery, and bell peppers through the juicer. Set aside ¼ cup each of the carrot, celery, and bell pepper juice. Combine the carrot, celery, and bell pepper pulps and set aside ½ cup.

2. In a medium-sized saucepan, combine the juices and pulp with the remaining ingredients and bring to a boil over high heat. Reduce the heat to medium-low and simmer uncovered for 15 minutes.

3. Strain the soup stock through a fine colander or cheesecloth, collecting the liquid.

4. Serve hot as is, or use as a base for other soups.

*Makes 1 Serving*

# Vegetable Millet Soup

1 recipe Classic Vegetable Stock (see page 139)

2 cups mineral water

½ zucchini, chopped

¼ cup chopped celery

¼ cup peeled and chopped carrot

⅛ cup millet

1. In a medium-sized saucepan, combine the stock with the mineral water and bring to a boil over high heat.

2. Reduce the heat to medium-low, add the remaining ingredients, and simmer uncovered for 10 minutes.

3. Serve hot with whole grain bread.

*Makes 2 Servings*

# Pasta and White Bean Soup

3 cucumbers (1½ cups juice)

½ head cauliflower, steamed and chilled (½ cup pulp)

¼ cup diced yellow onion

3 tablespoons extra virgin olive oil

¾ cup mineral water

1½ cups chopped tomatoes

¾ cup cooked white beans

½ cup chopped escarole or kale

¼ cup chopped celery

¼ cup peeled and chopped carrot

¼ cup uncooked whole grain macaroni

2 teaspoons chopped fresh parsley

2 teaspoons chopped fresh basil

½ teaspoon sea salt

½ teaspoon black pepper

1 clove garlic, crushed

1. Separately push the cucumbers and cauliflower through the juicer. Set aside 1½ cups of the cucumber juice and ½ cup of the cauliflower pulp.

2. In a large saucepan, sauté the onion in the oil 2–3 minutes.

3. Add the cucumber juice and mineral water and bring to boil over high heat. Reduce the heat to medium-low, add the remaining ingredients, and simmer uncovered for about 15 minutes, or until the pasta is tender.

4. Serve hot or cold with bread.

*Makes 2–4 Servings*

# Gingery Bean Soup

2 acorn squash, peeled, seeded, and cubed (1 cup juice
    and ½ cup pulp)

1 small piece ginger root (1 teaspoon juice)

2¾–3 cups mineral water

1 cup chopped tomatoes

¼ cup cooked white beans

1 tablespoon chopped fresh cilantro

¼ teaspoon sea salt

⅛ teaspoon black pepper

1. Separately push the squash and ginger through the juicer. Set aside 1 cup of the squash juice, ½ cup of the squash pulp, and 1 teaspoon of the ginger juice.

2. In a medium-sized saucepan, combine the juices and pulp with the remaining ingredients and bring to a boil over high heat. Reduce the heat to medium-low and simmer uncovered for 5–10 minutes.

3. Serve hot with whole grain bread.

*Makes 2 Servings*

# Gingery Carrot Soup

10 medium carrots, peeled, sliced lengthwise,
   tops removed

1 piece ginger root, cut into thirds (about 2-inch
   squares)

1 large lime, peeled, plus 1 large lime, sliced into
   quarters

1 large Vidalia onion, peeled and finely chopped (about
   2 cups)

10 large cloves garlic, peeled and pressed

1 tablespoon plus 1 teaspoon grated ginger

½ cup extra virgin olive oil

1½ teaspoons sea salt

freshly ground black pepper to taste (optional)

2 cups mineral water

⅓ cup plain nondairy yogurt

2 tablespoons finely chopped cilantro

1. Push the carrots, ginger, and the peeled lime through the juicer. Collect 1 cup of the carrot pulp and all of the carrot juice and set aside.

2. In a medium-sized saucepan, sauté the onion, garlic, and ginger in the oil over moderate heat for 7–8 minutes. When the onion becomes translucent, stir in the carrot juice mixture, carrot pulp, salt, pepper, if desired, and mineral water. Simmer partially covered for 10 minutes.

3. Serve hot or chilled, garnished with a dollop of yogurt, a sprinkling of cilantro, and a lime wedge.

*Makes 6–7 Cups*

# Mushroom Barley Soup

8 celery stalks (2 cups juice)

1 cup sliced leeks

2 tablespoons extra virgin olive oil

5½ cups mineral water

2 cups sliced mushrooms

1 cup chopped zucchini

½ cup pearl barley

1½ tablespoons chopped fresh dill

1½ teaspoons sea salt

1½ teaspoons black pepper

2 sprigs fresh dill, as garnish (optional)

1. Push the celery through the juicer. Set aside 2 cups of the juice.

2. In a large saucepan, sauté the leeks in the oil until soft.

3. Add the juice, mineral water, mushrooms, zucchini, barley, dill, salt, and pepper, and bring to a boil over high heat. Reduce the heat to medium-low and simmer uncovered for 25–35 minutes, or until the barley is done.

4. Serve hot, garnished with the dill sprigs, if desired.

*Makes 2 Servings*

# Celery Potato Soup

1 potato, steamed and chilled (½ cup juice and
   ½ tablespoon pulp)

2 celery stalks (½ cup juice)

¼ cup chopped leeks

½ cup cubed potatoes

1 tablespoon cold-pressed flavorless safflower oil

1¼ cups unsweetened soy milk

½ teaspoon finely chopped fresh dill

1 teaspoon finely chopped fresh parsley

¼ teaspoon celery seeds

½–¾ teaspoon sea salt

¼–½ teaspoon black pepper

2 sprigs fresh dill, as garnish (optional)

1. Separately juice the potato and celery. Set aside ½ cup of the potato juice, ½ tablespoon of the potato pulp, and ½ cup of the celery juice.

2. In a large saucepan, sauté the leeks and potato cubes in the oil for 3–4 minutes.

3. Add the juices, pulp, soy milk, dill, parsley, celery seeds, salt, and pepper, and bring to a boil over high heat. Reduce the heat to medium-low and simmer uncovered for about 10 minutes, or until the potatoes are tender.

4. Serve hot, garnished with the dill sprigs, if desired.

*Makes 2 Servings*

# Creamy Tomato Soup

1 butternut squash, peeled, seeded, and cubed
   (½ cup pulp)
½ tomato (¼ cup juice)
¼ cup plus 3 tablespoons plain soy yogurt, plus 2
   tablespoons plain soy yogurt, as garnish (optional)
¾ cup chopped tomatoes
2 teaspoons chopped fresh dill
¼ teaspoon sea salt
¼ teaspoon black pepper
2 tablespoons soy Parmesan cheese, as garnish
   (optional)
2 sprigs fresh dill, as garnish (optional)

1.  Separately push the squash and tomato through the juicer.
    Set aside ½ cup of the squash pulp and ¼ cup of the tomato
    juice.

2.  In a medium-sized saucepan, combine the pulp, juice, and
    yogurt. Bring to a simmer over medium-low heat and cook
    uncovered for 10–15 minutes.

3.  Add the chopped tomato, dill, salt, and pepper and remove
    from the heat.

4.  Serve hot or cold, garnished with the yogurt, Parmesan
    cheese, and dill sprigs, if desired.

*Makes 2 Servings*

# Oriental Miso Vegetable Soup

1 leek (¼ cup juice)

3 carrots peeled, sliced lengthwise, tops removed
    (¾ cup juice)

2 tablespoons brown rice miso

4 cups mineral water

½ cup destemmed shiitake mushrooms

1 cup diced extra-firm tofu

¼ cup snow pea pods

¼ cup peeled, seeded, and cubed squash (any type)

1 tablespoon toasted (dark) sesame oil

1 tablespoon chopped scallions

1 teaspoon chopped garlic

1 teaspoon chopped fresh cilantro

½ teaspoon grated ginger root

½ teaspoon diced red chili peppers

½ teaspoon hot (spicy) sesame oil

1.  Separately push the leek and carrots through the juicer. Set aside ¼ cup of the leek juice and ¾ cup of the carrot juice.

2.  In a large saucepan, dissolve the miso in the mineral water and stir well.

3.  Add the juices and remaining ingredients and bring to a boil over high heat. Reduce the heat to medium-low and simmer uncovered for 15–20 minutes.

4.  Serve hot with whole grain bread.

*Makes 2 Servings*

# Southwestern Squash Soup

1 butternut squash, peeled, seeded, and cubed
(1 cup juice)

¼ cup cooked black beans

¼ cup mineral water

2 tablespoons plain soy yogurt, plus 2 tablespoons plain
soy yogurt, as garnish (optional)

½ cup chopped tomatoes, plus 2 tablespoons chopped
tomatoes, as garnish (optional)

1 teaspoon chopped fresh basil, or ½ teaspoon dried
basil

½ teaspoon finely chopped jalapeño peppers

½ teaspoon finely chopped fresh cilantro

2 sprigs fresh cilantro, as garnish (optional)

1. Push the squash through the juicer. Set aside 1 cup of the juice.

2. In a blender or food processor, combine the black beans with the mineral water and blend until you have a smooth purée. Set aside ½ cup of the purée.

3. In a medium-sized saucepan, combine the squash juice, black bean purée, and 2 tablespoons yogurt. Mix thoroughly with a whisk until creamy.

4. Add the ½ cup tomatoes, basil, jalapeño peppers, and chopped cilantro and simmer uncovered over medium-low heat for 5–10 minutes.

5. Serve hot or cold, garnished with 2 tablespoons yogurt, 2 tablespoons tomatoes, and cilantro sprigs, if desired.

*Makes 2 Servings*

# Summer Cool Gazpacho

8 large tomatoes, quartered

1 large yellow bell pepper, cored, seeded, and finely
    chopped (about 1⅓ cups)

1 medium Vidalia onion, peeled and finely chopped
    (about 1 cup)

2 tablespoons finely chopped parsley (flat-leafed
    preferred) or cilantro

4 large cloves garlic, peeled and pressed

¼ cup freshly squeezed lemon juice (about 1 large
    lemon)

5 tablespoons extra virgin olive oil

2 teaspoons sea salt

freshly ground black pepper to taste (optional)

⅓ cup plain nondairy yogurt, as garnish (optional)

⅓ cup cherry tomatoes, halved, as garnish (optional)

⅓ cup packed thinly sliced fresh basil leaves, as
    garnish (optional)

1. Push 4 tomatoes through the juicer. Set aside all of the tomato juice. Dice the remaining 4 tomatoes into ¼-inch cubes.

2. In a large bowl, combine the diced tomatoes, yellow pepper,
   onion, parsley, and garlic. Drizzle the tomato juice, lemon
   juice, and olive oil onto the vegetables and gently toss together until well coated. Sprinkle with salt and black pepper,
   if desired. Toss again.

3. Serve chilled, garnished with a dollop of yogurt, a few cherry
   tomatoes, and basil leaves, if desired.

*Makes 10 Servings*

# Chilled Cucumber Mint Soup

2 cucumbers (1 cup juice), plus ½ cup chopped peeled
     cucumbers

4 celery stalks (1 cup juice)

1 cup plain nondairy yogurt

2 teaspoons finely chopped fresh mint

2 teaspoons chopped fresh parsley

¼ cup diced red bell pepper or pomegranate seeds, as
     garnish (optional)

2 sprigs fresh mint, as garnish (optional)

1.  Separately push the 2 cucumbers and celery through the
    juicer. Set aside 1 cup of the cucumber juice and 1 cup of the
    celery juice.

2.  In a medium-sized mixing bowl, combine the juices, yogurt,
    chopped cucumber, mint, and parsley. Blend with a whisk un-
    til creamy. Chill for one hour.

3.  Serve cold, garnished with the diced red peppers and mint
    sprigs, if desired.

*Makes 2 Servings*


# Papaya Squash Soup

2–3 acorn squash, peeled, seeded, and cubed
     (1¼ cups juice and ½ cup pulp)

2 papayas, peeled, pitted, and quartered (1 cup juice),
     plus ¼ cup papaya slices, as garnish (optional)

2½–3 cups mineral water

½ teaspoon ground nutmeg

¼ cup halved seedless red grapes or pomegranate
     seeds, as garnish (optional)

1. Separately push the squash and the 2 papayas through the juicer. Set aside 1¼ cups of the squash juice, ½ cup of the squash pulp, and 1 cup of the papaya juice.

2. In a medium-sized saucepan, combine the juices, pulp, mineral water, and nutmeg and bring to a boil over high heat. Reduce the heat to medium-low and simmer uncovered for 5–7 minutes.

3. Serve hot or cold, garnished with the papaya slices and red grapes, if desired.

*Makes 2 Servings*

# Cold Cherry Soup

2 cups pitted cherries
1 lemon, peeled and quartered
1 cup strawberries, hulled
1 cup blueberries
¼ cup agar-agar
ground cinnamon to taste, as garnish (optional)
1 orange, sliced into wedges, as garnish (optional)

1. Push the cherries and lemon through the juicer.

2. Blend the strawberries, blueberries, and agar-agar with the juice mixture until well combined.

3. Serve in a bowl, and garnish with cinnamon and orange wedges, if desired.

*Makes 2 Cups*

# Cinnamon Fruit Soup

1 butternut squash, peeled, seeded, and cubed
    (½ cup juice and ¾ cup pulp)
2 pears, cored and quartered (½ cup juice)
1½ cups unsweetened soy milk
1 teaspoon pure vanilla extract
¾ teaspoon ground cinnamon
6 slices orange, as garnish (optional)
2 sprigs fresh mint, as garnish (optional)

1.  Separately push the squash and pears through the juicer. Set aside ½ cup of the squash juice, ¾ cup of the squash pulp, and ½ cup of the pear juice.

2.  In a medium-sized saucepan, combine the juices, pulp, soy milk, vanilla extract, and cinnamon and bring to a boil over high heat. Reduce the heat to medium-low and simmer uncovered for 4–6 minutes.

3.  Serve hot or cold, garnished with the orange slices and mint sprigs, if desired.

*Makes 2 Servings*

# Papaya Nectar Soup

4 small papayas, peeled, pitted, and cut into 2-inch
    pieces (about 8 cups)
16 large nectarines, pitted and quartered
4 large limes, peeled
⅓ cup lemon-flavored nondairy yogurt
fresh mint sprigs, as garnish (optional)

1.  Push the papayas, nectarines, and limes through the juicer.
    Stir the juice well.

2.  Serve chilled in bowls with a dollop of yogurt and garnished
    with mint sprigs (2 per bowl), if desired.

*Makes 1 Gallon*

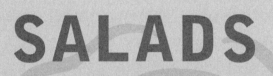

# SALADS

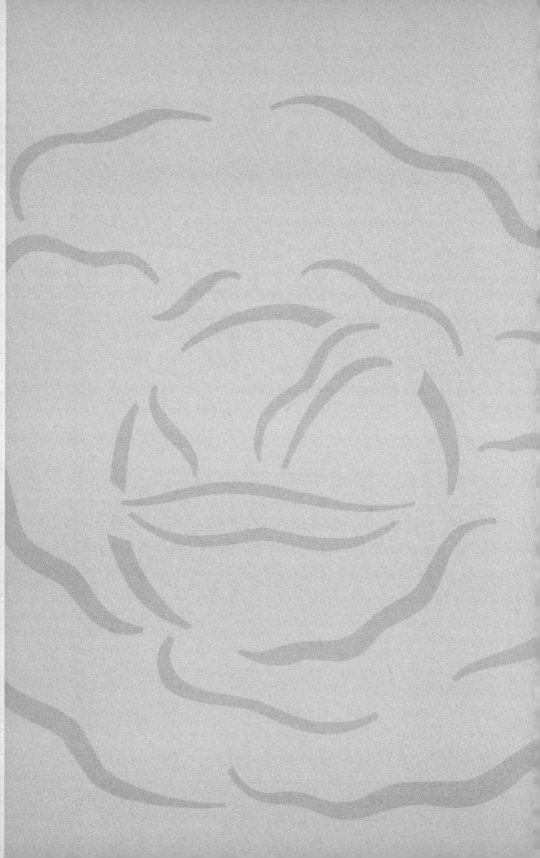

# Curried Waldorf Salad

½ lemon, peeled and quartered (1 tablespoon juice)

2 cups diced unpeeled apples, seeded

2 cups diced unpeeled pears, seeded

1 cup diced celery

1 cup unsalted walnut halves

½ cup raisins

½ cup Curry Mayonnaise (see page 193)

1. Push the lemon through the juicer. Set aside 1 tablespoon of the juice.

2. In a medium-sized mixing bowl, combine the lemon juice with the remaining ingredients and mix well.

3. Serve chilled or at room temperature.

*Makes 2 Servings*

# A Chef's Salad

1 head fresh, young romaine lettuce

1 head butter lettuce (about 1½ pounds)

1 recipe Creamy Italian Dressing (see page 180)

2 cups Savory Croutons (see page 162)

1 recipe "Bacon Bits" (see page 159)

4 ounces Vidalia onion, thinly sliced

⅓ cup black olives, pitted

1. Trim the base of the lettuce and discard any bruised outer leaves. Use the tender inner leaves, keeping the small leaves whole and cutting or tearing the larger outer leaves crosswise into halves or thirds. Wash and dry the greens in a spinner and transfer to a large bowl.

2. Toss the salad with the desired amount of Creamy Italian Dressing until well coated. Toss briefly with the croutons, "Bacon Bits," onion, and olives, and serve immediately.

*Makes 12 Servings*

# "Bacon Bits"

1 pound extra-firm tofu, crumbled

¾ cup extra virgin olive oil

1 large clove garlic, peeled and finely chopped

1 teaspoon dried marjoram

1 teaspoon rubbed sage

1 teaspoon dried basil

¼ teaspoon dried oregano

½ teaspoon sea salt

freshly ground black pepper to taste (optional)

1.  Preheat the broiler. Line an 11-by-15-inch cookie sheet with parchment paper and set aside.

2.  In a medium-sized mixing bowl, toss together the tofu, oil, garlic, marjoram, sage, basil, oregano, salt, and black pepper, if desired.

3.  Evenly spread the seasoned tofu on the prepared cookie sheet and broil in the preheated oven for about 15 minutes, or until golden. For uniformity in broiling, rotate the sheet from front to back halfway through the baking period.

4.  Remove the sheet from the oven and cool the bits completely.

5.  Toss with salads.

*Makes 3 Servings*

# Caesar Salad with Thyme Croutons

3 carrots, peeled, sliced lengthwise, tops removed
(¾ cup pulp)

4½ cups chopped romaine lettuce

¼ cup Dijon Salad Dressing (see page 180)

¾ cup Thyme Croutons (see below)

1½ tablespoons grated soy Parmesan cheese

1. Push the carrots through the juicer. Set aside ¾ cup of the pulp.

2. In a large mixing bowl, toss the carrot pulp with the lettuce.

3. Toss the salad with Dijon Salad Dressing, Thyme Croutons, and soy Parmesan cheese, and serve cold or at room temperature.

*Makes 2 Servings*

# Thyme Croutons

1 cup whole grain ¾-inch bread cubes

2–4 tablespoons extra virgin olive oil

1½ tablespoons finely chopped fresh thyme

dash of sea salt

1. Preheat the oven to 375°F.

2. In a small mixing bowl, combine all the ingredients and toss.

3. Spread the cubes on an ungreased 11-by-15-inch cookie sheet and bake for 15–20 minutes, or until light brown in color.

4. Toss with salads.

*Makes 1 Cup*

# Insalata Caesar

2 heads fresh, young romaine lettuce (about 1½ pounds)

1 recipe Creamy Caesar Dressing (see page 179)

2 cups Savory Croutons (see page 162)

4 sheets julienne strips of sushi nori

1. Trim the base of the romaine lettuce and discard any bruised outer leaves. Use the tender inner leaves, keeping the small leaves whole and cutting or tearing the larger outer leaves crosswise into halves or thirds. Wash and dry the greens in a spinner and transfer to a large bowl.

2. Toss the desired amount of Creamy Caesar Dressing onto the salad greens until well coated. Toss briefly with the croutons, top with nori, and serve immediately.

*Makes 4 Servings*

# Savory Croutons

2 cups cut-up millet or rice bread, cut into ¾-inch cubes

2 tablespoons extra virgin olive oil

1 tablespoon grated soy Parmesan-style nondairy

  cheese

¼ teaspoon dried basil

¼ teaspoon dried marjoram

¼ teaspoon dried oregano

sea salt to taste

1. Preheat the oven to 425°F. Line an 11-by-15-inch cookie sheet with parchment paper and set aside.

2. In a medium-sized mixing bowl, toss together the bread, oil, cheese, basil, marjoram, oregano, and salt. Evenly spread the seasoned cubes on the prepared cookie sheet and bake in the preheated oven for 8–10 minutes, or until golden. For uniformity in baking, rotate the sheet front to back halfway through the baking period. Remove the sheet from the oven and cool the croutons completely.

3. Toss with salads.

*Makes 2 Cups*

# Mixed Dark Green Salad

2 beets (½ cup pulp)

1 cup chopped radicchio

1 cup chopped Belgian endive

1 cup chopped arugula

1 cup chopped Swiss chard

1 cup unsalted walnut halves

1 recipe Dijon Salad Dressing (see page 180)

1.  Push the beets through the juicer. Set aside ½ cup of the pulp.

2.  In a large mixing bowl, toss the beet pulp with the radicchio, endive, arugula, Swiss chard, and walnuts.

3.  Toss the salad with the desired amount of Dijon Salad Dressing and serve cold or at room temperature with whole grain bread.

*Makes 2 Servings*

# Mixed Sprout Salad

2 beets (½ cup pulp)

2 cups lentil sprouts

1 cup radish sprouts

1 cup alfalfa sprouts

1 cup sliced red bell peppers

1 recipe Sesame Orange Dressing (see page 182)

1. Push the beets through the juicer. Set aside ½ cup of the pulp.

2. In a large mixing bowl, toss the beet pulp with the sprouts and bell peppers.

3. Toss the salad with the desired amount of Sesame Orange Dressing and serve at room temperature.

*Makes 2 Servings*

# Cucumber Raita Salad

½ cucumber (¼ cup juice), plus ½ cup chopped peeled
   cucumbers
2 cups plain soy yogurt
1 tablespoon chopped fresh cilantro
2 teaspoons ground cardamom
½ cup chopped tomatoes

1.  Push the ½ cucumber through the juicer. Set aside ¼ cup of
    the juice.

2.  In a small mixing bowl, combine the cucumber juice with the
    yogurt and mix well with a whisk.

3.  Stir in the cilantro and cardamom and mix.

4.  Add the chopped cucumbers and tomatoes and mix.

5.  Serve cold or at room temperature with bread or almost any
    main dish. This salad goes especially well with Matar Paneer
    (see page 207).

*Makes 2 Servings*

# Green Bean Salad with Almonds and Dill

    2 cups steamed green beans

    ¼ cup Dill Mayonnaise (see page 192)

    ¼ cup slivered blanched almonds

    1 tablespoon poppy seeds

    ¼ cup fresh dill sprigs, as garnish (optional)

1.  In a medium-sized mixing bowl, toss the beans with the Dill Mayonnaise.

2.  Sprinkle the almonds and poppy seeds on top of the bean mixture.

3.  Serve cold or at room temperature, garnished with the dill sprigs, if desired.

*Makes 1 Serving*


# Red Potato Salad

    ½ carrot, peeled, sliced lengthwise, top removed
        (1 tablespoon juice and 2 tablespoons pulp)

    2 cups diced steamed red potatoes

    ½ cup chopped celery

    2 tablespoons chopped red onions

    2 tablespoons extra virgin olive oil

    2 teaspoons chopped fresh dill

    1 teaspoon celery seeds

    1 teaspoon sea salt

    ½ teaspoon black pepper

    ⅛–¼ cup soy mayonnaise

1.  Push the carrot through the juicer. Set aside 1 tablespoon of the juice and 2 tablespoons of the pulp.

2. In a medium-sized mixing bowl, toss the carrot juice and pulp with the remaining ingredients.

3. Serve cold or at room temperature.

*Makes 2 Servings*

# Coleslaw with Fresh Dill

1 carrot, peeled, sliced lengthwise, top removed (¼ cup pulp)

2 lemons, peeled and quartered (3 tablespoons juice)

2 cups shredded green cabbage

3 tablespoons soy mayonnaise

½ teaspoon prepared mustard

1 tablespoon chopped fresh dill

½ teaspoon sea salt

¼ teaspoon black pepper

dash of apple cider vinegar

1. Separately push the carrot and lemons through the juicer. Set aside ¼ cup of the carrot pulp and 3 tablespoons of the lemon juice.

2. In a medium-sized mixing bowl, toss the carrot pulp and lemon juice with the remaining ingredients.

3. Serve cold as a salad or a sandwich filling.

*Makes 2 Servings*

# Tomato Garlic Pasta Salad

4 cups cooked whole grain pasta (bow ties, shells,
   or ziti)

3 cups Tomato Salsa (see page 190)

2 cups steamed broccoli florets

1 cup whole pine nuts

1. In a large mixing bowl, toss the pasta with the remaining ingredients.

2. Serve cold as a main dish or a salad.

*Makes 2 Servings*

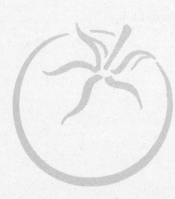

# Beach Salad

3–4 heads fresh, young mixed lettuces (Bibb, endive, and
  radicchio) (about 1½ pounds)
1 recipe Mixed Citrus Vinaigrette (see page 181)
1 large carrot, peeled and grated
1 large beet, peeled and grated
1 large yellow bell pepper, cored, seeded, and finely
  chopped
1 five-ounce fennel bulb, thinly sliced
1 recipe Heavenly Roasted Nuts (see page 131)

1. Trim the base of the lettuces and discard any bruised outer leaves. Use the tender inner leaves, keeping the small leaves whole and thinly slicing the larger outer leaves into crosswise strips. Wash and dry the greens in a spinner and transfer to a large bowl.

2. Drizzle the desired amount of Mixed Citrus Vinaigrette onto the lettuces, carrot, beet, yellow pepper, and fennel to taste and gently toss together until well coated. Toss briefly with the nuts and serve immediately.

*Makes 12 Servings*

# Tabouli Salad

1 cup boiling mineral water

3 cups bulghur wheat

3 carrots, peeled, sliced lengthwise, tops removed
   (¾ cup pulp)

2 lemons (¼ cup juice)

½ cup raisins

½ cup finely chopped fresh parsley

½ cup chopped unsalted cashews

¼ cup sliced scallions

2–3 tablespoons tamari soy sauce

1.  In a large mixing bowl, pour the boiling mineral water over the bulghur wheat. Cover the bowl with a towel and let it stand for 30 minutes. Drain off any excess liquid.

2.  Separately push the carrots and lemons through the juicer. Set aside ¾ cup of the carrot pulp and ¼ cup of the lemon juice.

3.  In a large mixing bowl, combine the carrot pulp, lemon juice, and bulghur wheat with the remaining ingredients. Mix well and drain off any excess liquid.

4.  Serve cold or at room temperature with whole grain bread.

*Makes 2 Servings*

# Nature's Total Salad

2 heads fresh, young romaine lettuce (about 1½ pounds)

½ pound sunflower sprouts

1 recipe Lemon Garlic Dressing (see page 181)

2 ripe Hass avocados, peeled, halved, pitted, and sliced

1 large cucumber, halved, seeded, and thinly sliced

1 cup cooked millet

½ cup unsalted roasted cashews

1. Trim the base of the lettuces and discard any bruised outer leaves. Use the tender inner leaves, keeping the small leaves whole and cutting or tearing the larger outer leaves crosswise into halves or thirds. Wash and dry the greens and sunflower sprouts in a spinner and transfer to a large bowl.

2. Drizzle the desired amount of Lemon Garlic Dressing onto the lettuce, sprouts, avocados, cucumber, and millet and gently toss together until well coated. Toss briefly with the cashews and serve immediately.

*Makes 4–5 Servings*

# Succotash Salad

About 4 quarts mineral water

1 twelve-ounce package quinoa macaroni

2 large Vidalia onions, peeled and thinly sliced

½ cup extra virgin olive oil

1 small kuri squash, peeled, seeded, and
chopped into ¾-inch pieces (about 2 cups)

½ pound extra-firm tofu (crumbled)

1 ten-ounce package frozen lima beans

2 cups fresh corn kernels (about 3–4 ears)

1 six-ounce can pitted black olives, sliced

1 large red bell pepper, cored, seeded, and diced

4 large celery stalks, finely chopped

½ cup chopped parsley (curly leafed preferred)

½ cup freshly squeezed lemon juice

1 tablespoon plus 1 teaspoon sea salt

1 tablespoon dried basil

freshly ground black pepper to taste (optional)

sweet relish to taste

paprika, as garnish (optional)

1. In a large pot, bring the mineral water to a rolling boil. Stir the macaroni into the water and cook until the pasta is just tender but not soft, 4–5 minutes. Transfer to a colander, drain, and place in a large mixing bowl to cool.

2. While the pasta is cooking, in a large saucepan sauté the onions in the oil over moderate heat for 6–8 minutes, or until tender. Remove the onions from the heat and gently toss into the cooked pasta, until well coated.

3. Place the kuri squash pieces on a steamer set into a large pot filled with 1 inch of mineral water. Cook covered over moderate to high heat until the squash is tender when a fork is

inserted into its center, about 8 minutes. Remove the squash from the steamer and gently toss into the macaroni mixture.

4. Add the tofu, lima beans, and corn to the steamer and cook covered for 10 minutes, or until the lima beans are hot. Remove the tofu, lima beans, and corn from the steamer and gently toss into the macaroni mixture.

5. Add the olives, bell pepper, celery, parsley, lemon juice, salt, basil, black pepper, if desired, and relish to the macaroni and gently toss together until well coated. Serve warm or chilled, garnished with a sprinkling of paprika, if desired.

*Makes 4–5 Servings*

# Tempeh "Turkey" Salad

1 twelve-ounce package three-grain tempeh, crumbled

About 4 quarts mineral water

½ cup sunflower seeds

2 large carrots, peeled, sliced lengthwise, tops removed
   (¾ cup pulp)

1 large stalk celery, finely chopped

¼ cup finely chopped onion

¼ cup finely chopped parsley (curly leafed preferred)

2 large cloves garlic, peeled and finely chopped

¼ cup soy mayonnaise

2 tablespoons extra virgin olive oil

2 tablespoons freshly squeezed lemon juice (about ½
   lemon)

1 tablespoon plus 1 teaspoon sea salt

1 tablespoon plus 1 teaspoon tamari soy sauce

1 teaspoon dried basil

freshly ground black pepper to taste (optional)

paprika, as garnish (optional)

1.  Place the tempeh on a steamer set into a large pot filled with
    1 inch of mineral water. Cook covered over moderate to high
    heat until the tempeh is tender when a fork is inserted into
    its center, about 10 minutes. Remove the tempeh from the
    steamer and transfer to a large mixing bowl.

2.  While the tempeh is cooking, in a small saucepan sauté the
    sunflower seeds over moderate heat for 4–5 minutes, or until
    golden. Remove from the heat and gently toss into the tempeh
    mixture until well combined.

3.  Add the carrot pulp, celery, onions, parsley, garlic, soy mayon-
    naise, olive oil, lemon juice, salt, tamari, basil, and black pep-

per, if desired. Gently toss together until well coated. Serve warm or chilled, garnished with a sprinkling of paprika, if desired.

*Makes 4 Servings*

# Summer Fruit Salad

½ apple, cored and halved (2 teaspoons juice)

½ lemon, peeled and halved (1½ teaspoons juice)

1 cup peeled, diced peaches

½ cup blueberries

½ cup strawberries

½ cup raspberries

½ teaspoon pure almond extract

1.  Separately push the apple and lemon through the juicer. Set aside 2 teaspoons of the apple juice and 1½ teaspoons of the lemon juice.

2.  In a medium-sized mixing bowl, combine the juices with the remaining ingredients and mix well.

3.  Serve cold.

*Makes 2 Servings*

# Blackberry Nectarine Fruit Salad

1 large cantaloupe, rind removed, seeded and cut into
   1-inch pieces (about 4 cups)

8 large nectarines, pitted and sliced (about 4 cups)

4 cups blackberries

1 tablespoon freshly squeezed lemon juice

3 tablespoons freshly squeezed lime juice

2 tablespoons powdered brown rice syrup (optional)

1.  In a large bowl, combine the cantaloupe, nectarines, and blackberries.

2.  Drizzle the lemon juice and lime juice onto the fruit and gently toss together until well coated.

3.  Spoon into small bowls, sprinkle with powdered brown rice syrup, if desired, and serve.

*Makes 4–6 Servings*

# DRESSINGS, SAUCES, DIPS, AND SPREADS

# Creamy Caesar Dressing

¼ cup extra virgin olive oil

¼ cup mineral water

¼ cup tahini

¼ cup silken tofu

¼ cup freshly squeezed lemon juice (about 1 large
   lemon)

1 teaspoon tamari soy sauce

2 tablespoons chopped parsley

1 large clove garlic, peeled and finely chopped

¼ teaspoon dried basil

¼ teaspoon paprika

¼ teaspoon sea salt

1. Blend the oil, mineral water, tahini, tofu, lemon juice, soy
   sauce, parsley, garlic, basil, paprika, and salt on medium
   speed for 3 minutes, or until smooth and creamy.

2. Serve over salads.

*Makes About 1¼ Cups*

# Creamy Italian Dressing

1 cup silken tofu

½ cup extra virgin olive oil

½ cup freshly squeezed lemon juice (about 2 large
lemons)

¼ cup chopped parsley

2 large cloves garlic, peeled and finely chopped

16 fresh basil leaves

½ teaspoon sea salt

freshly ground black pepper to taste (optional)

1. Blend the tofu, oil, lemon juice, parsley, garlic, basil, salt, and
pepper, if desired, on medium speed for 3 minutes, or until
smooth and creamy.

2. Serve over salads.

*Makes About 2 Cups*


# Dijon Salad Dressing

¾ cup cold-pressed flavorless safflower oil

6 tablespoons mineral water

3 tablespoons prepared Dijon mustard

3 tablespoons apple cider vinegar

1 teaspoon finely chopped fresh herbs (chives, basil,
and/or parsley)

¼ teaspoon sea salt

¼ teaspoon black pepper

1. In a small mixing bowl, combine all the ingredients and mix
well with a fork or whisk.

2. Serve over salads.

*Makes 1 Cup*

# Lemon Garlic Dressing

½ cup extra virgin olive oil

½ cup freshly squeezed lemon juice (about 2 large
  lemons)

¼ cup chopped parsley

2 large cloves garlic, peeled and finely chopped

2 teaspoons sea salt

freshly ground black pepper to taste (optional)

1. Blend the oil, lemon juice, parsley, garlic, salt, and pepper, if desired, in a blender on medium speed until well combined.

2. Serve over salads.

*Makes About 1¼ Cups*


# Mixed Citrus Vinaigrette

¼ cup extra virgin olive oil

¼ cup freshly squeezed lemon juice (1 large lemon)

¼ cup freshly squeezed lime juice (1 large lime)

¼ cup freshly squeezed orange juice (1 large orange)

sea salt to taste

freshly ground black pepper to taste (optional)

1. Blend the oil, lemon juice, lime juice, orange juice, salt, and black pepper, if desired, in a blender on medium speed until well combined.

2. Serve over salads.

*Makes 1 Cup*

# Sesame Orange Dressing

3 oranges, peeled and quartered (¾ cup juice)

¼ cup toasted (dark) sesame oil

3 tablespoons sesame seeds

2 tablespoons hot (spicy) sesame oil

1.  Push the oranges through the juicer. Set aside ¾ cup of the juice.

2.  In a small mixing bowl, combine the orange juice with the remaining ingredients and mix well.

3.  Serve cold or at room temperature over salads.

*Makes 1¼ Cups*


# Tomato Salad Dressing

1 tomato (½ cup juice)

2 lemons, peeled and quartered (3 tablespoons juice)

½ cup extra virgin olive oil

1 teaspoon chopped fresh basil, or ½ teaspoon dried basil

½ teaspoon chopped fresh oregano, or ¼ teaspoon dried oregano

1 clove garlic, crushed

1.  Separately push the tomato and lemons through the juicer. Set aside ½ cup of the tomato juice and 3 tablespoons of the lemon juice.

2.  In a blender or food processor, combine the juices with the remaining ingredients and blend for about 2 minutes, or until smooth.

3.  Serve at room temperature over salads.

*Makes 1¼ Cups*

# Sunflower Salad Dressing

2 lemons, peeled and quartered (¼ cup juice)

¼ cup unsalted hulled sunflower seeds

½ cup extra virgin olive oil

½ cup soft tofu

1–2 tablespoons mineral water

1 tablespoon tamari soy sauce

1 teaspoon chopped fresh basil, or ½ teaspoon dried
   basil

1 teaspoon chopped fresh thyme, or ½ teaspoon dried
   thyme

1. Push the lemons through the juicer. Set aside ¼ cup of the juice.

2. Grind the sunflower seeds in a food mill or food processor.

3. In a blender or food processor, combine the lemon juice and ground sunflower seeds with the remaining ingredients, and blend for about 2 minutes, or until smooth.

4. Serve cold over salads or with raw vegetables.

*Makes 1¼ Cups*

# Cilantro Mint Dressing

4 lemons, peeled and quartered (½ cup juice)

1 cup finely chopped fresh cilantro

3 tablespoons mineral water

1½ tablespoons finely chopped fresh mint

1½ teaspoons finely chopped green chili peppers

1. Push the lemons through the juicer. Set aside ½ cup of the juice.

2. In a small mixing bowl, combine the lemon juice with the remaining ingredients and mix well.

3. Serve cold over salads. This dressing is especially good with Cucumber Raita Salad (see page 165) and unleavened bread.

*Makes 1½ Cups*

# Tahini Garbanzo Bean Dressing

2 lemons, peeled and quartered (3 tablespoons juice)

⅛ cup cooked garbanzo beans (chickpeas)

2 tablespoons mineral water

¼ cup sesame tahini

1 clove garlic, crushed

¼ teaspoon sea salt

1. Push the lemons through the juicer. Set aside 3 tablespoons of the juice.

2. In a blender or food processor, combine the garbanzo beans and mineral water and blend until you have a smooth purée. Set aside 1 cup of the purée.

3. In a small mixing bowl, combine the lemon juice and garbanzo bean purée with the remaining ingredients and blend with a whisk until smooth.

4. Serve at room temperature over salads, vegetables, brown rice, or whole grain pasta.

*Makes 1¼ Cups*

# Zesty Tomato Sauce

2 tomatoes (1 cup juice), plus 2½ cups chopped
   tomatoes
¼ cup chopped green bell peppers
2 tablespoons chopped yellow onion
¼ cup extra virgin olive oil
1 tablespoon tomato paste
1 tablespoon finely chopped fresh basil
1 clove garlic, crushed
½ teaspoon sea salt
½ teaspoon black pepper

1. Push the 2 tomatoes through the juicer. Set aside 1 cup of the juice.

2. In a medium-sized saucepan, sauté the bell peppers and onions in the oil for 5 minutes.

3. Add the tomato juice, the chopped tomatoes, and the remaining ingredients and simmer over medium-low heat for 15–20 minutes.

4. Serve hot over whole grain pasta.

*Makes 4 Cups*

# Cilantro Pesto Sauce

1 large bunch fresh parsley (¾ cup pulp, plus juice)

1 small bunch fresh cilantro (¼ cup pulp, plus juice)

2 tablespoons ground or whole unsalted walnuts or
   walnut butter

½ cup extra virgin olive oil

1 clove garlic, minced

½ teaspoon sea salt

½ teaspoon black pepper

1.  Separately push the parsley and cilantro through the juicer. Set aside ¾ cup of the parsley pulp and ¼ cup of the cilantro pulp. Combine the parsley and cilantro juices and set aside 1 tablespoon.

2.  In a blender or food processor, combine the parsley pulp, cilantro pulp, and mixed juices with the remaining ingredients and blend for about 2 minutes, or until smooth.

3.  Serve at room temperature over vegetables or whole grain pasta.

*Makes 1 Cup*


# Curried Orange Sauce

1 orange, peeled and quartered (¾ cup juice)

⅛ cup cooked garbanzo beans (chickpeas)

2 tablespoons mineral water

1 teaspoon curry powder

¼ teaspoon sea salt

1.  Push the orange through the juicer. Set aside ¼ cup of the juice.

2.  In a blender or food processor, combine the garbanzo beans

and mineral water and blend until you have a smooth purée. Set aside 1 cup of the purée.

3.   In a small mixing bowl, combine the orange juice and garbanzo bean purée with the remaining ingredients and blend with a whisk until smooth.

4.   Serve hot or cold over vegetables, brown rice, or whole grain pasta.

*Makes 1¼ Cups*

# Walnut Pesto Sauce

1 large bunch fresh parsley (¾ cup pulp, plus juice)
1 small bunch fresh basil (¼ cup pulp, plus juice)
2 tablespoons ground or whole unsalted walnuts or
    walnut butter
½ cup extra virgin olive oil
1 clove garlic, minced
½ teaspoon sea salt
½ teaspoon black pepper

1.   Separately push the parsley and basil through the juicer. Set aside ¾ cup of the parsley pulp and ¼ cup of the basil pulp. Combine the parsley and basil juices, and set aside 1 tablespoon.

2.   In a blender or food processor, combine the parsley pulp, basil pulp, and mixed juices with the remaining ingredients and blend for about 2 minutes, or until smooth.

3.   Serve at room temperature over vegetables or whole grain pasta.

*Makes 1 Cup*

# Guacamole and Bermuda Onion Dip

2 lemons, peeled and quartered (3 tablespoons juice)

4 sprigs fresh cilantro (1 tablespoon pulp)

1 cup mashed avocado

¼ cup silken tofu

¼ teaspoon finely chopped jalapeño peppers

¼ teaspoon sea salt

¼ cup finely chopped red Bermuda onions

¼ cup finely chopped tomatoes

1. Separately push the lemons and cilantro through the juicer. Set aside 3 tablespoons of the lemon juice and 1 tablespoon of the cilantro pulp.

2. In a blender or food processor, combine the lemon juice, cilantro pulp, avocado, tofu, jalapeño peppers, and salt and blend for about 2 minutes, or until smooth.

3. Transfer the mixture to a small mixing bowl, add the remaining ingredients, and mix well with a spoon.

4. Serve cold or at room temperature with raw vegetables or corn chips.

*Makes 1¾ Cups*


# Tangy Carrot Dip

½ carrot peeled, sliced lengthwise, top removed
   (2 tablespoons juice)

¾ cup soft tofu

½ cup cubed or mashed steamed sweet potatoes

2 tablespoons apple cider vinegar

¼ teaspoon ground cinnamon

1. Push the carrot through the juicer. Set aside 2 tablespoons of the juice.

2. In a blender or food processor, combine the carrot juice with the remaining ingredients and blend for about 2 minutes, or until smooth.

3. Serve cold with raw vegetables.

*Makes 1½ Cups*

# Lemony Hummus

5 lemons, peeled and quartered (½ cup plus
   2 tablespoons juice)
1 clove garlic (½ teaspoon pulp)
1½ cups sesame tahini
1 cup cooked garbanzo beans (chickpeas)
¼ cup mineral water
½ teaspoon sea salt

1. Separately push the lemons and garlic through the juicer. Set aside ½ cup plus 2 tablespoons of the lemon juice, and ½ teaspoon of the garlic pulp.

2. In a blender or food processor, combine the lemon juice and garlic pulp with the remaining ingredients and blend for about 2 minutes, or until smooth.

3. Serve cold or at room temperature with raw vegetables or on bread.

*Makes 3 Cups*

# Tomato Salsa

6 leaves fresh basil (1½ tablespoons pulp)

2 cups chopped tomatoes

¼ cup extra virgin olive oil

1 tablespoon crushed garlic

1 teaspoon sea salt

½ teaspoon black pepper

1. Push the basil through the juicer. Set aside 1½ tablespoons of the pulp.

2. In a small mixing bowl, combine the basil pulp with the remaining ingredients and mix.

3. Serve cold or at room temperature with corn chips, on toast, or over whole grain pasta.

*Makes 2¼ Cups*

# Sweet Kidney Bean Mash

1 pound sweet potatoes or yams, scrubbed well and cut into 2-inch-thick slices (about 2 cups)

¼ cup extra virgin olive oil

1 eight-ounce yellow onion, peeled and finely chopped

2 large celery stalks, finely chopped

3 large cloves garlic, peeled and coarsely chopped

1 pound cooked kidney beans, rinsed and drained

¼ cup freshly squeezed lime juice

10 large basil leaves

1 teaspoon sea salt

¾ teaspoon ground cumin

¼ teaspoon ground chili powder

freshly ground black pepper to taste (optional)

8 slices of whole grain country bread or millet bread, cut
½ inch thick

1. Place the sweet potato slices onto a steamer set into a large
   pot filled with 1 inch of water. Cook covered over moderate to
   high heat until the potatoes are tender when a fork is inserted
   into their centers, 15–20 minutes. Remove the steamer and
   run the potatoes under cool water until they can be handled
   comfortably. Using a small paring knife, remove and discard
   the peels.

2. In a medium-sized saucepan, combine the oil, onion, celery,
   and garlic. Sauté over moderate heat for 5–7 minutes, or until
   the onions are translucent.

3. In a food processor, using a metal blade, combine the sautéed
   vegetables with the sweet potatoes, kidney beans, lime juice,
   basil leaves, salt, cumin, chili powder, and black pepper, if
   desired. Process together until smooth and creamy, about 2
   minutes. Set aside.

4. Lightly toast the bread on both sides. Spread the bread slices
   with the sweet mash and serve warm.

*Makes 4–6 Servings*

# Basil Mayonnaise

1 large bunch fresh basil (½ cup pulp)
2 cloves garlic (1 teaspoon pulp)
1½ cups soy mayonnaise

1. Separately push the basil and garlic through the juicer. Set aside ½ cup of the basil pulp and 1 teaspoon of the garlic pulp.

2. In a blender or food processor, combine the basil and garlic pulp with the soy mayonnaise and blend for about 2 minutes, or until smooth. Keep refrigerated in a covered glass jar.

3. Serve with raw vegetables.

*Makes 2 Cups*

# Dill Mayonnaise

1 large bunch fresh dill (½ cup pulp)
½ lemon (2 teaspoons juice)
1½ cups soy mayonnaise

1. Separately push the dill and lemon through the juicer. Set aside ½ cup of the dill pulp and 2 teaspoons of the lemon juice.

2. In a blender or food processor, combine the dill pulp and lemon juice with the soy mayonnaise and blend for about 2 minutes, or until smooth. Keep refrigerated in a covered glass jar.

3. Serve with raw vegetables.

*Makes 2 Cups*

# Curry Mayonnaise

¾ teaspoon ground cumin

¾ teaspoon ground turmeric

¼ teaspoon mustard powder

¼ teaspoon ground ginger

⅛ teaspoon ground cinnamon

⅛ teaspoon cayenne pepper

1½ cups soy mayonnaise

1.  In a blender or food processor, combine all the ingredients and blend for 2 minutes, or until smooth. Keep refrigerated in a covered glass jar.

2.  Serve with raw vegetables.

*Makes 1½ Cups*

# Orange Apricot Spread

12 oranges, peeled and quartered (3 cups juice and ¼
   cup pulp)
½ cup chopped dried apricots
¼ cup finely chopped orange peel
¼ cup chopped dates
2 tablespoons apple cider vinegar
1 tablespoon finely chopped red onion
dash of ground allspice

1. Push the oranges through the juicer. Set aside 3 cups juice and ¼ cup pulp.

2. In a medium-sized saucepan, bring the orange juice to a boil over high heat.

3. Reduce the heat to medium-low, add the remaining ingredients, and simmer for 15–20 minutes, or until the mixture reaches the consistency of spreadable preserves. Remove from the heat and let cool before using.

4. Serve cold or at room temperature with breads and muffins.

*Makes 2 Cups*

# Cranberry Chutney

12 apples, cored and quartered (3 cups juice and ½ cup
   pulp)
1 cup cranberries
½ cup chopped dried apricots
4 tablespoons chopped dates
2 tablespoons apple cider vinegar
2 tablespoons diced red onion
¼ teaspoon ground allspice

1. Push the apples through the juicer. Set aside 3 cups of the juice and ½ cup of the pulp.

2. In a small saucepan, bring the apple juice to a boil over high heat.

3. Reduce the heat to medium-low, add the remaining ingredients, and simmer for 15–20 minutes, or until the mixture reaches the consistency of spreadable preserves. Remove from the heat and let cool before using.

4. Serve cold or at room temperature with any vegetable dish.

*Makes 2 Cups*

# Peanut Butter Honey Spread

½ peeled banana, frozen (¼ cup pulp)

1 cup unsalted peanuts

3 tablespoons light-colored honey (clover, tupelo, or wildflower)

1. Push the frozen banana through the juicer. Set aside ¼ cup of the pulp (mashed banana).

2. In a blender, food processor, or food mill, blend the peanuts until they are smooth and creamy.

3. In a small mixing bowl, combine the banana pulp, peanut butter, and honey until well mixed.

4. Serve at room temperature with breads and muffins or fresh fruit slices.

*Makes 1¼ Cups*

# Basil Herb Oil

4 leaves fresh basil (1 tablespoon pulp)

2 cloves garlic (1 teaspoon pulp)

9 tablespoons extra virgin olive oil

¼ teaspoon sea salt

1.  Separately push the basil and garlic through the juicer. Set aside 1 tablespoon of the basil pulp and 1 teaspoon of the garlic pulp.

2.  In a small mixing bowl, combine the basil and garlic pulp with the remaining ingredients and blend with a whisk until smooth.

3.  Serve at room temperature with breads and muffins, or toss with hot whole grain pasta.

*Makes ½ Cup*

# MAIN
# DISHES

# Fettuccine with Pesto and Tomatoes

1 cup sliced mushrooms

1 cup broccoli florets

3 tablespoons extra virgin olive oil

3 cups cooked whole grain fettuccine

1 recipe Walnut Pesto Sauce (see page 187)

1 cup chopped tomatoes

¼ cup grated soy Parmesan cheese, as garnish
(optional)

1. In a large saucepan, sauté the mushrooms and broccoli in the oil over high heat for 3–5 minutes.

2. Reduce the heat to low, add the fettuccine and Walnut Pesto Sauce, and toss.

3. Add the tomatoes and toss.

4. Serve hot, garnished with soy cheese, if desired.

*Makes 2 Servings*

# Mushroom Lasagna

4 carrots, peeled, sliced lengthwise, tops removed
  (1 cup pulp)

4 cups soy ricotta cheese

vegetarian egg substitute for 2 eggs

½ cup grated soy Parmesan cheese

¼ cup chopped fresh parsley

½ teaspoon sea salt

¼ teaspoon black pepper

2 cups broccoli florets

2 cups sliced mushrooms

3 tablespoons extra virgin olive oil

2 cups Zesty Tomato Sauce (see page 185)

1 pound cooked whole grain lasagna noodles

3½ cups shredded soy mozzarella cheese

1. Preheat the oven to 425°F.

2. Push the carrots through the juicer. Set aside 1 cup of the pulp.

3. In a medium-sized mixing bowl, combine the carrot pulp, soy ricotta cheese, egg substitute, soy Parmesan cheese, parsley, salt, and pepper, and mix well with a whisk. Set aside.

4. In a large saucepan, sauté the broccoli and mushrooms in the oil over high heat for 3–5 minutes. Set aside.

5. Spread 1 cup of the Zesty Tomato Sauce on the bottom of an ungreased 12-by-17-inch lasagna pan or baking dish. On top of the sauce, arrange a layer of lasagna noodles, a layer of broccoli and mushrooms, a layer of the soy ricotta mixture, a layer of soy mozzarella cheese, and another layer of noodles. Repeat the layers, ending with additional layers of sauce and soy mozzarella.

6. Cover the lasagna and bake for 45–55 minutes. Let stand for 7 minutes before cutting.

7. Serve hot with a salad and whole grain bread.

*Makes 6–8 Servings*

# Zesty Italian Pizza

1 cup chopped plum tomatoes with juice

1 packed cup chopped fresh basil

¼ cup chopped sun-dried tomatoes

1 tablespoon Cilantro Pesto Sauce (see page 186)

½ teaspoon sea salt

2 pieces whole wheat pita bread

¾ cup shredded soy mozzarella cheese

½ cup grated soy Parmesan cheese

1. Preheat the oven to 350°F.

2. In a small mixing bowl, combine the plum tomatoes, basil, sun-dried tomatoes, Cilantro Pesto Sauce, and salt, and mix well.

3. Place the pita bread on an ungreased 11-by-15-inch cookie sheet and spread with the tomato mixture. Sprinkle the top of each pizza with the soy mozzarella and soy Parmesan cheese.

4. Bake the pizzas for 15–20 minutes, or until the tops are bubbly.

5. Serve hot with a salad.

*Makes 2 Servings*

# Mushroom Broccoli Quiche

1 tomato (½ cup juice)

1 large bunch fresh basil (½ cup pulp)

1 cup silken tofu

1 cup Guacamole and Bermuda Onion Dip (see page 188)

¾ cup grated soy Parmesan cheese

2 tablespoons extra virgin olive oil

⅛ teaspoon sea salt

⅛ teaspoon black pepper

1¼ cups thinly sliced broccoli

1¼ cups thinly sliced mushrooms

1 recipe Basic Spelt Crust, prebaked (see page 220)

1. Preheat the oven to 375°F.

2. Separately push the tomato and basil through the juicer. Set aside ½ cup of the tomato juice and ½ cup of the basil pulp.

3. In a blender or food processor, combine the tomato juice, basil pulp, tofu, Guacamole and Bermuda Onion Dip, soy cheese, oil, salt, and black pepper and blend for about 1 minute, or until creamy.

4. Arrange the broccoli and mushrooms on the bottom of the prepared Basic Spelt Crust. Pour the tofu mixture over the vegetables.

5. Bake the quiche uncovered for 25–30 minutes, or until the top of the quiche has set and begun to turn light brown in color. Remove the quiche from the oven and let stand for 5 minutes before cutting.

6. Serve hot with a salad.

*Makes 6–8 Servings*

# Spicy Texas Chili

4 carrots, peeled, sliced lengthwise, tops removed
    (1 cup juice)

3 red or green bell peppers, cored, seeded, and
    quartered (¼ cup juice), plus ¼ cup chopped green
    bell peppers

½ cup finely chopped yellow onion

¼ cup extra virgin olive oil

½ eggplant, chopped

½ cup cooked garbanzo beans (chickpeas)

½ cup cooked red kidney beans

½ cup sliced pattypan squash or zucchini

⅓ cup stewed tomatoes

¼ cup corn kernels, fresh or frozen

¼ cup tomato purée

2½ teaspoons chopped green chili peppers

1 clove garlic, crushed

1. Separately push the carrots and the 3 bell peppers through the juicer. Set aside 1 cup of the carrot juice and ¼ cup of the pepper juice.

2. In a large saucepan, sauté the onion in the oil over high heat until the onion is soft, about 3 minutes.

3. Add the remaining ingredients to the saucepan and bring to a boil. Reduce the heat to medium-low and simmer uncovered for 15–20 minutes, or until the vegetables are tender.

4. Serve hot with spelt bread or whole grain pasta.

*Makes 2 Servings*

# Curried Red Lentil Stew

2 carrots, peeled, sliced lengthwise, tops removed
  (½ cup juice)

2 stalks celery (½ cup juice)

1 beet (¼ cup juice)

¼ cup finely chopped yellow onion

2 tablespoons extra virgin olive oil

½ cup finely chopped tomatoes

3¾ cups mineral water

¾ cup dried red lentils

1½ tablespoons finely chopped fresh cilantro

1 teaspoon dried parsley

1 teaspoon dried basil

¾ teaspoon curry powder

1 bay leaf

dash of ground cardamom

1¼ cups assorted frozen vegetables (carrots, broccoli,
  and/or cauliflower)

1.  Separately push the carrots, celery, and beet through the juicer. Set aside ½ cup of the carrot juice, ½ cup of the celery juice, and ¼ cup of the beet juice.

2.  In a large saucepan, sauté the onion in the oil over high heat until soft, about 3 minutes.

3.  Reduce the heat to medium-low. Add the juices, tomatoes, mineral water, and lentils and cook uncovered for 15 minutes.

4.  Add the cilantro, parsley, basil, curry powder, bay leaf, and cardamom and cook for an additional 25 minutes.

5. Add the frozen vegetables and cook, stirring occasionally, for another 15 minutes, or until the vegetables are tender and the lentils are done. Remove bay leaf and discard.

6. Serve hot with brown rice.

*Makes 2 Servings*

# Lentil Burgers

4 carrots, peeled, sliced lengthwise, tops removed

   (½ cup pulp)

1 cup cooked red lentils

¼ cup lentil sprouts

¼ cup ground unsalted cashews or cashew butter

2 tablespoons chopped unsalted almonds

1 tablespoon diced yellow onions

2 teaspoons curry powder

½ teaspoon ground coriander

½ teaspoon sea salt

½ cup whole spelt bread crumbs

1. Preheat the oven to 425°F.

2. Push the carrots through the juicer. Set aside ½ cup of the pulp.

3. In a small mixing bowl, combine the carrot pulp with the lentils, lentil sprouts, cashews, almonds, onions, curry powder, coriander, and salt and mix well.

4. Shape the mixture into 2 patties, coat the patties with the bread crumbs, and place them on an ungreased 11-by-15-inch cookie sheet.

5. Bake the patties for 10 minutes, turn the patties over, and bake for an additional 10–15 minutes.

6. Serve hot in pita bread pockets with Lemony Hummus (see page 189).

*Makes 2 Servings*

# Matar Paneer

1 tomato, quartered (½ cup juice)

16 ounces extra-firm tofu, cut into 1-inch cubes

2 tablespoons safflower oil

¾ cup chopped yellow onions

2 cups frozen peas

1 cup chopped tomatoes

¾ cup unsweetened soy milk

3 teaspoons apple cider vinegar

½ cup finely chopped fresh cilantro

2 fresh green chili peppers, finely chopped

3 cloves garlic, crushed

2 teaspoons grated ginger root

1 teaspoon ground coriander

1 teaspoon ground turmeric

¼ teaspoon chili powder

1½ teaspoons sea salt

1. Push the tomato through the juicer. Set aside ½ cup of the juice.

2. In a large frying pan, brown the tofu in the oil over high heat.

3. Add the onions and sauté for 2–3 minutes, or until the onions are soft.

4. Reduce the heat to medium-low, add the remaining ingredients, and simmer uncovered for an additional 5 minutes.

5. Serve hot with Peas Pillau with Cinnamon (see page 212).

*Makes 4 Servings*

# Stir-Fried Broccoli with Tempeh and Lemon Threads

5 cups fresh basil (1 cup pulp)

1 small bunch fresh cilantro (¼ cup pulp)

2 lemons, peeled and quartered (¼ cup juice), plus
   1 lemon

2 cloves garlic (1 teaspoon pulp)

¼ cup tamari soy sauce

1–2 tablespoons whole grain flour

1 tablespoon apple cider vinegar

1 teaspoon chopped red chili peppers

1 teaspoon grated ginger root

2 cups tempeh, cut into 1-inch cubes

¼ cup toasted (dark) sesame oil

2½ cups broccoli florets

¼ cup sliced scallions

1 pint cherry tomatoes

1.  Separately push the basil, cilantro, 2 lemons, and garlic through the juicer. Set aside 1 cup of the basil pulp, ¼ cup of the cilantro pulp, ¼ cup of the lemon juice, and 1 teaspoon of the garlic pulp.

2.  Peel the remaining lemon, and slice the peel into threads. Set aside 1 tablespoon of the threads.

3.  In a blender or food processor, combine the basil, cilantro, and garlic pulp with the lemon juice, soy sauce, flour, vinegar, peppers, and ginger and blend for 2 minutes.

4.  Transfer the basil mixture to a small saucepan, stir in the lemon peel threads, and heat for 4–5 minutes, or until warm.

5.  In a large frying pan, brown the tempeh in the oil over medium to high heat.

6. Reduce the heat to medium-low, add the broccoli and scallions, cover, and cook for 2 minutes.

7. Add the tomatoes and cook uncovered for 1 additional minute.

8. Arrange the tempeh mixture on a serving platter and pour the heated sauce over the mixture.

9. Serve hot with brown rice.

*Makes 2–3 Servings*

# Scalloped Autumn Vegetables

10 parsnips, cubed (½ cup juice and 2 tablespoons pulp)

1½ cups unsweetened soy milk

2 tablespoons chopped fresh parsley

1 tablespoon cold-pressed flavorless safflower oil

½ teaspoon sea salt

1 teaspoon chopped fresh thyme, or ½ teaspoon dried
thyme

¼ teaspoon chopped fresh rosemary, or ¼ teaspoon
dried rosemary

1 clove garlic, crushed

1½ cups sliced parsnips

1 cup sliced white potatoes

1 cup acorn squash, peeled, seeded, and sliced

½ cup chopped leeks

2 cups grated soy mozzarella cheese (optional)

1. Preheat the oven to 425°F.

2. Push the parsnips through the juicer. Set aside ½ cup of the juice and 2 tablespoons of the pulp.

3. In a small mixing bowl, combine the parsnip juice and pulp, soy milk, parsley, oil, salt, thyme, rosemary, and garlic and mix well.

4. In a medium-sized mixing bowl, toss together the sliced parsnips, potatoes, squash, and leeks.

5. Arrange the vegetables on the bottom of a greased 9-by-13-inch baking dish or other large glass or ceramic dish. Pour the sauce over the vegetables and sprinkle on the cheese, if desired. Cover with a glass lid or aluminum foil and bake for 25 minutes, or until the vegetables are tender.

6. Serve hot with a salad or whole grain pasta.

*Makes 4 Servings*

# Zesty Cauliflower with Garlic and Tahini

1 recipe Tahini Garbanzo Bean Dressing (see page 184)

1 cup cauliflower florets

1 cup broccoli florets

1 cup sliced red bell peppers, plus ½ cup diced red bell pepper, as garnish (optional)

½ cup unsalted whole cashews

4 sprigs fresh parsley, as garnish (optional)

1. Preheat the oven to 425°F.

2. In a medium-sized mixing bowl, combine the Tahini Garbanzo Bean Dressing, cauliflower, broccoli, sliced bell peppers, and cashews and toss to mix.

3. Pour the mixture into a greased 9-by-13-inch baking dish or other large glass or ceramic dish. Cover with a glass lid or aluminum foil and bake for 25–35 minutes, or until the cauliflower is tender. (The other vegetables should still be crunchy.)

4. Garnish with the diced bell peppers and parsley, if desired, and serve hot or cold with any rice or pasta dish.

*Makes 2 Servings*

# Peas Pillau with Cinnamon

4 carrots, peeled, sliced lengthwise, tops removed
   (1 cup juice)

2 teaspoons saffron threads

2 teaspoons mineral water, plus 2 cups mineral water

1 cup uncooked white Basmati rice

3 tablespoons sesame oil

1½ cups frozen peas

1 tablespoon ground cardamom

1 stick cinnamon

1 teaspoon sea salt

½ teaspoon black pepper

1. Push the carrots through the juicer. Set aside 1 cup of the juice.

2. Dissolve the saffron threads in the 2 teaspoons of mineral water.

3. In a medium-sized saucepan, sauté the rice in the oil over medium to high heat until the rice is light brown in color, about 4 minutes.

4. Add the carrot juice, saffron, and 2 cups of mineral water, and bring the mixture to a boil over high heat. Reduce the heat to medium-low, cover, and cook for 12–15 minutes, or until all of the water is absorbed.

5. Stir in the remaining ingredients and continue cooking until the mixture is hot.

6. Remove the cinnamon stick and serve hot with Matar Paneer (see page 207) or a salad and whole grain bread.

*Makes 2–4 Servings*

# Japanese Rice with Shiitake Mushrooms

2-inch piece ginger root (2 tablespoons juice)

1½ cups sliced destemmed shiitake mushrooms

1 cup sliced zucchini

3 tablespoons safflower or other light oil

1 cup mung bean sprouts, drained

½ cup tamari soy sauce

3 teaspoons sliced scallions

4 cups cooked short-grain brown rice

1. Push the ginger through the juicer. Set aside 2 tablespoons of the juice.

2. In a large frying pan, sauté the mushrooms and zucchini in the oil over high heat until soft.

3. Reduce the heat to medium-low. Add the ginger juice, bean sprouts, soy sauce, and scallions and simmer for 1–2 minutes, or until the mixture has thickened.

4. Spoon the vegetable mixture over the rice and serve hot.

*Makes 2 Servings*

# DESSERTS

# Sweet Potato Pie

1 apple, cored and quartered (¼ cup juice)

3 cups mashed steamed sweet potatoes

vegetarian egg substitute for 2 eggs

¼ cup pure maple syrup

1½ teaspoons ground allspice

1 recipe Basic Spelt Crust, prebaked (see page 220)

1. Preheat the oven to 350°F.

2. Push the apple through the juicer. Set aside ¼ cup of the juice.

3. In a blender or food processor, combine the apple juice, sweet potatoes, egg substitute, maple syrup, and allspice and blend until smooth.

4. Pour the sweet potato mixture into the prepared pie crust and bake for 25 minutes, or until the crust is golden and the filling is set.

5. Allow the pie to cool for 10 minutes before serving.

*Makes One 9-Inch Pie*

# Apple Pecan Cobbler

## FILLING

> 2 pears, cored and quartered (½ cup juice and ¾ cup
>    pulp)
>
> 2 apples, cored and quartered (½ cup juice and ¾ cup
>    pulp), plus 3½ cups sliced apples, unpeeled
>
> 1 orange, peeled and quartered (¼ cup juice)
>
> ½ lemon, peeled (1 tablespoon juice)
>
> ½ teaspoon ground cinnamon
>
> ⅔ cup chopped apricots (dried or fresh)

## TOPPING

> 3 cups coarsely chopped unsalted pecans
>
> 1 cup coarsely chopped unsalted macadamia nuts
>
> 1 cup pure maple syrup
>
> 3 tablespoons safflower oil
>
> 2 teaspoons pure almond extract
>
> 1 teaspoon grated orange peel
>
> 2 teaspoons ground cinnamon
>
> ¼ cup chopped dates

1. Preheat the oven to 400°F.

2. Separately push the pears, the 2 apples (not the slices), the orange, and the lemon through the juicer. Set aside ½ cup of the pear juice and ¾ cup of the pear pulp, ½ cup of the apple juice and ¾ cup of the apple pulp, ¼ cup of the orange juice, and 1 tablespoon of the lemon juice.

3. In a medium-sized mixing bowl, combine the apple slices with the pear, apple, and orange juices. Stir in the pear and apple pulp, lemon juice, ½ teaspoon of cinnamon, and apricots, mixing well.

4. In another medium-sized mixing bowl, combine all the topping ingredients except the dates and 1 teaspoon of the cinnamon, mixing well.

5. In a small mixing bowl, combine the dates with the remaining 1 teaspoon of cinnamon and mix well.

6. Pour the apple slice mixture into a greased 9-by-13-inch baking dish, spreading the filling evenly so that it touches all sides of the pan.

7. Pour the topping over the filling and spread it evenly with a knife.

8. Bake the cobbler for 30–35 minutes, or until the apples are soft. Remove from the oven, and sprinkle with the cinnamon and dates mixture.

9. Serve hot or cold with rice or soy ice cream.

*Makes 6–8 Servings*

# Basic Spelt Crust

1 cup whole spelt flour

½ teaspoon ground cinnamon

4 tablespoons extra virgin olive oil

¼ cup plus 3 tablespoons cold mineral water or
   unsweetened soy milk

1.  In a small mixing bowl, combine the whole spelt flour and cinnamon.

2.  With a fork or pastry cutter, mix the olive oil into the flour mixture until the mixture is moist and fine. Add the cold mineral water (or soy milk) by the tablespoon until the dough has a smooth, even consistency.

3.  Roll the dough into a ball and place it in a bowl. Cover the bowl with plastic wrap and chill for 1 hour.

4.  Flour a smooth, clean surface and a rolling pin with all-purpose flour. Place the chilled dough on the floured surface and roll the dough from the center out until it is ½ inch larger than a 9-inch pie plate. (Check by placing the empty pie plate on top of the rolled dough.)

5.  Loosen the dough by gently sliding a floured spatula underneath it toward the center and moving around the entire area of the dough until it can be lifted. Transfer the dough to a lightly greased 9-inch pie plate.

6.  When a recipe calls for a baked crust, put the crust in a 350°F oven for 15 minutes, or until light brown in color.

*Makes One 9-Inch Crust*

# Sweet Potato Crust

4 sweet potatoes, steamed and chilled (2 cups pulp)

vegetarian egg substitute for 1 egg

¼ cup finely chopped dates

½ teaspoon pure almond extract

1.  Preheat the oven to 350°F.

2.  Push the sweet potatoes through the juicer. Set aside 2 cups of
    the pulp.

3.  In a small mixing bowl, combine the sweet potato pulp, egg
    substitute, dates, and almond extract and mix together well.

4.  Press the mixture into a lightly greased 9-inch pie plate and
    bake for 40 minutes, or until golden brown in color.

*Makes One 9-Inch Crust*

# Date Nut Crust

3 parsnips, cubed (½ cup pulp)

3 cups whole pitted dates

1½ cups unsalted pecans, soaked for 24 hours and
drained

1.  Push the parsnips through the juicer. Set aside ½ cup of the pulp.

2.  In a blender or food processor, combine the parsnip pulp, dates, and pecans and blend until smooth.

3.  Press the mixture into a lightly greased 9-inch pie plate.

4.  When a recipe calls for a baked crust, put the crust in a 350°F oven for 15 minutes, or until light brown in color.

*Makes One 9-Inch Crust*

# A Sunny Day Crust

 1 cup unsalted roasted cashews

 ⅓ cup yellow cornmeal

 ⅓ cup quinoa flour

 ⅓ cup unsweetened coconut

 a pinch of sea salt

 ¼ cup extra virgin olive oil

 ¼ cup freshly squeezed lemon juice

 1 teaspoon honey (optional)

1.  Preheat the oven to 325°F. Lightly oil and flour a 13-by-4-by-1½-inch tart pan with a removable bottom and set aside.

2.  In a food processor, using the metal blade, process the cashews until they are powder-fine. Add the cornmeal, flour, coconut, and salt and process until well combined. Restart the food processor and slowly add the oil, lemon juice, and honey, if desired, through the feed tube. Process until soft and crumbly.

3.  Transfer the mixture to the prepared pan and distribute evenly. Press and shape the dough into the pan to form an even crust.

4.  Place the tart pan on top of an 11-by-15-inch cookie sheet and bake in the preheated oven for 25–30 minutes, or until golden. For uniformity in baking, rotate the sheet from front to back halfway through the baking period. Remove the sheet from the oven, transfer to a wire rack, and cool completely.

*Makes 1 Crust*

# Banana Almond Bread

1 peeled banana, frozen (½ cup pulp)

vegetarian egg substitute for 1 egg

½ cup light-colored honey (clover, tupelo, or wildflower)

⅓ cup cold-pressed flavorless oil (sunflower or
safflower)

1 teaspoon pure almond extract

1¼ cups plus 1 tablespoon whole spelt flour

1 teaspoon baking soda

½ teaspoon ground nutmeg

½ teaspoon ground cinnamon

¼ teaspoon sea salt

½ cup mineral water

¼ cup slivered blanched almonds

1. Preheat the oven to 350°F.

2. Push the frozen banana through the juicer. Set aside ½ cup of
   the pulp (mashed banana).

3. In a medium-sized mixing bowl, combine the egg substitute,
   honey, oil, and almond extract.

4. In a small mixing bowl, sift together the flour, baking soda,
   nutmeg, cinnamon, and salt.

5. Add a small amount of the flour mixture to the egg substitute mixture and blend well. Then add a small amount of
   the mineral water to the egg substitute mixture and blend
   well. Alternate adding the remaining flour mixture and the
   water to the egg mixture, making sure to blend well after each
   addition.

6. Add the banana and almonds to the batter and mix well with
   a sturdy spoon.

7. Pour the batter into a greased 3-by-7-inch loaf pan. Bake

for 15 minutes, remove the loaf from the oven, and make a 1-inch-deep slice lengthwise down the center of the loaf (this facilitates cooking the center). Return the loaf to the oven, and bake for an additional 25–30 minutes, or until a toothpick inserted in the center comes out clean.

8. Allow the bread to cool for 5 minutes before removing it from the pan. Cool the bread for at least 5 additional minutes before slicing.

*Makes One 3-by-7-Inch Loaf*

# Gingerbread

1 small piece ginger root (¼ teaspoon juice and ¼
   teaspoon pulp)

⅓ cup safflower oil

½ cup light-colored honey (tupelo, clover, or wildflower)

⅓ cup unsulfured blackstrap molasses

vegetarian egg substitute for 1 egg

¼ cup chopped dates

½ cup unsweetened soy milk

¼ cup mineral water

1¾ cups plus 1 tablespoon whole spelt flour

1 teaspoon baking powder

½ teaspoon ground cinnamon

¼ teaspoon ground nutmeg

¼ teaspoon sea salt

1 recipe Cocoa Coconut Frosting (see page 227)

1. Preheat the oven to 350°F.

2. Push the ginger through the juicer. Set aside ¼ teaspoon of the juice and ¼ teaspoon of the pulp.

3. In a medium-sized mixing bowl, combine the ginger juice and pulp, oil, honey, molasses, egg substitute, dates, soy milk, and mineral water. Stir the ingredients well.

4. In a small mixing bowl, sift together the flour, baking powder, cinnamon, nutmeg, and salt. Add to the oil mixture and blend well.

5. Grease the bottom of a 9-inch round or 10-inch square baking pan, line with parchment paper, and regrease. Pour the batter into the pan and bake for 15–20 minutes, or until a toothpick inserted in the center of the cake comes out clean.

6. Allow the cake to cool for 5 minutes before removing it from

the pan. Remove the parchment paper and cool completely before glazing with Cocoa Coconut Frosting.

*Makes One 9-Inch Cake*

### Cocoa Coconut Frosting

¾ cup light-colored honey (clover, tupelo, or wildflower)

¼ cup plus 2 tablespoons pure unsweetened cocoa powder (unsweetened carob powder may be substituted)

3 tablespoons plain soy yogurt (optional)

1 teaspoon pure almond extract

2 tablespoons unsweetened flaked coconut

1. In a small mixing bowl, whisk together all of the ingredients except the coconut until a smooth frosting is formed.

2. Add the coconut and mix well.

*Makes 1 Cup*

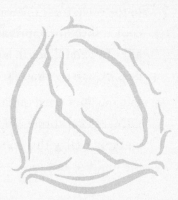

# Pumpkin and Spice Muffins

1 sweet potato, steamed and chilled (½ cup juice)

½ small pumpkin, rind removed, seeded and cubed
(¾ cup pulp)

¾ cup unsalted walnut halves

vegetarian egg substitute for 2 eggs

½ cup plus 2 tablespoons cold-pressed flavorless
oil (sunflower or safflower)

½ cup chopped dates

1 banana, mashed

1 teaspoon pure vanilla extract

2 cups stone-ground whole spelt flour

1 teaspoon baking powder

1 teaspoon baking soda

1 teaspoon ground nutmeg

½ teaspoon ground allspice

½ teaspoon ground cinnamon

½ cup raisins

1.  Preheat the oven to 350°F.

2.  Separately push the sweet potato and pumpkin through the juicer. Set aside ½ cup of the sweet potato juice (pumpkin juice may be substituted) and ¾ cup of the pumpkin pulp.

3.  In the oven, toast the walnuts on an ungreased 11-by-15-inch cookie sheet for approximately 10 minutes, stirring occasionally. (Be careful not to let them burn, as this causes bitterness.) Coarsely chop the nuts and set aside.

4.  In a medium-sized mixing bowl, combine the sweet potato juice, egg substitute, oil, dates, banana, and vanilla extract and mix well with a sturdy spoon. Add the pumpkin pulp to the mixture and stir.

5.   In a small mixing bowl, sift together the flour, baking powder, baking soda, nutmeg, allspice, and cinnamon.

6.   Add the flour mixture to the egg substitute mixture and blend well. Stir in the toasted nuts and raisins.

7.   Pour the batter into greased or paper-lined muffin tins and bake for 25–30 minutes, or until a toothpick inserted in the center of a muffin comes out clean.

*Makes 24 Muffins*

# Carrot Walnut Cake

2 oranges, peeled and quartered (½ cup juice)

2 sweet potatoes, steamed and chilled (1 cup juice)

6 carrots, peeled, sliced lengthwise, tops removed (1½
   cups pulp)

1½ cups unsalted walnut halves

¾ cup unsalted pecan halves

vegetarian egg substitute for 2 eggs

1 cup cold-pressed safflower flavorless oil

1 cup light-colored honey (clover, tupelo, or wildflower)

2 teaspoons pure almond extract

4½ cups stone-ground whole spelt flour

2¼ teaspoons baking powder

1¼ teaspoons baking soda

1 teaspoon ground cinnamon

½ teaspoon ground nutmeg

¼ teaspoon ground cloves

1 cup chopped dates

1. Preheat the oven to 350°F.

2. Separately push the oranges, sweet potatoes, and carrots through the juicer. Set aside ½ cup of the orange juice, 1 cup of the sweet potato juice (carrot juice may be substituted), and 1½ cups of the carrot pulp.

3. In the oven, toast the walnuts and pecans on an ungreased 11-by-15-inch cookie sheet for approximately 10 minutes, stirring occasionally. (Be careful not to let them burn, as this causes bitterness.) Coarsely chop the nuts and set aside.

4. In a medium-sized mixing bowl, combine the orange and sweet potato juices, egg substitute, oil, honey, and almond extract and mix well. Stir in the carrot pulp.

5. In a large mixing bowl, sift the flour with the baking powder, baking soda, cinnamon, nutmeg, and cloves.

6. Add the egg substitute mixture to the flour mixture and blend with an electric handheld mixer until smooth. Add the dates and toasted nuts to the batter and mix well.

7. Pour the batter into 2 greased 3-by-7-inch loaf pans and bake for 45 minutes to 1 hour, or until a toothpick inserted in the center of the loaves comes out clean.

8. Allow the loaves to cool for about 5 minutes before removing from the pans. Cool the loaves for at least 5 additional minutes before slicing.

*Makes Two 3-by-7-Inch Loaves*

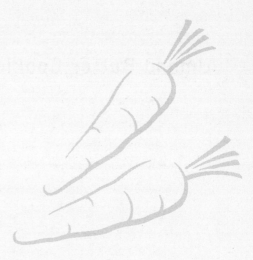

# Raspberry Crowned Lemon Tart

1 recipe for custard (any type without eggs or dairy)

juice of 2 lemons (freshly squeezed)

4 tablespoons honey

1 recipe prebaked A Sunny Day Crust (see page 223)

1 pint fresh raspberries

1 recipe Smooth Vanilla Sauce (see page 262)

1 recipe Red Raspberry Coulis (see page 262)

1. Combine the custard, lemon juice, and honey. Mix well.

2. To assemble the tart, pour the honey lemon custard into the baked tart shell and spread evenly. Then carefully distribute the berries on top.

3. Refrigerate for 60 minutes, or until well set and firm to the touch. Carefully push up the bottom and slide the tart off the disk and onto a cutting board.

4. Using a sharp knife, slice into 10–12 equal wedges and serve on dessert plates accompanied by a drizzling of Smooth Vanilla Sauce and Red Raspberry Coulis.

*Makes 1 Pie*

# Almond Butter Cookies

2–3 parsnips, cubed (⅓ cup pulp)

¼ cup almonds, plus ½ cup ground unsalted almonds or almond butter

4 tablespoons safflower oil

⅓ cup light-colored honey (clover, tupelo, or wildflower)

2 teaspoons pure almond extract

3 cups spelt flour

2 tablespoons baking powder

1 teaspoon sea salt

1½ teaspoons ground cinnamon

¼ cup chopped dates

1. Push the parsnips through the juicer. Set aside ⅓ cup of the pulp.

2. In the oven, toast the almonds on an ungreased 11-by-15-inch cookie sheet for approximately 10 minutes at 350°F, stirring occasionally. (Be careful not to let them burn, as this causes bitterness.) In a blender, food processor, or food mill, grind the nuts and set aside.

3. In a medium-sized mixing bowl, cream together the oil, honey, and almond extract.

4. In another medium-sized mixing bowl, sift together the flour, baking powder, salt, and 1 teaspoon of the cinnamon.

5. Add the flour mixture to the oil mixture and stir to blend. Stir in the ½ cup ground almonds (or almond butter) and the parsnip pulp, blending thoroughly with a sturdy spoon.

6. Roll the dough into a log and cover with plastic wrap. Chill for 1 hour.

7. Preheat the oven to 350°F.

8. In a small mixing bowl, combine the remaining ½ teaspoon of cinnamon with the dates and the ground toasted almonds.

9. Remove the cookie dough from the refrigerator. On a floured surface, roll the dough to ¼-inch thickness with a rolling pin and use cookie cutters to cut the dough into the desired shapes. Sprinkle the shapes with the cinnamon mixture and bake on an ungreased 11-by-15-inch cookie sheet for 10–15 minutes, or until the cookies are light brown along the edges.

*Makes 18 Cookies*

# Holiday Surprise Cookies

2 sweet potatoes, steamed and chilled (1 cup pulp)

1 cup unsalted pecan halves

1 cup unsalted walnut halves

vegetarian substitute for 2 eggs

1½ cups chopped dates

2 tablespoons pure maple syrup

½ cup safflower oil

1 teaspoon pure vanilla extract

1 teaspoon pure almond extract

1⅔ cups plus 2 tablespoons whole spelt flour

1 teaspoon baking soda

1 teaspoon baking powder

1 teaspoon ground cinnamon

½ teaspoon sea salt

1½ cups raisins

1 cup rolled oats

½ cup unsweetened carob chips

¼ cup unsweetened flaked coconut

¼ cup unsalted hulled sunflower seeds

1. Preheat the oven to 375°F.

2. Push the sweet potatoes through the juicer. Set aside 1 cup of the pulp.

3. In the oven, toast the pecans and walnuts on an ungreased 11-by-15-inch cookie sheet for approximately 10 minutes, stirring occasionally. (Be careful not to let them burn, as this causes bitterness.) Coarsely chop the nuts and set aside.

4. In a medium-sized mixing bowl, combine the sweet potato pulp, egg substitute, dates, maple syrup, safflower oil, and vanilla and almond extracts. Blend well with an electric hand-held mixer.

5. In a small mixing bowl, sift together the flour, baking soda, baking powder, cinnamon, and salt.

6. Add the flour mixture to the sweet potato mixture and blend well with a sturdy spoon. Stir in the toasted nuts, raisins, oats, carob chips, coconut, and sunflower seeds and mix well.

7. Roll the dough into 1-inch balls. Place the balls on an ungreased 11-by-15-inch cookie sheet and bake for about 15 minutes, or until the cookies turn light brown in color.

*Makes 24 Cookies*

# Fruit and Nut Cookies

1 carrot, peeled, sliced lengthwise, top removed
   (2 tablespoons pulp)
½ cup unsalted pecan halves
¾ cup whole unsalted almonds
vegetarian egg substitute for 1 egg
3 tablespoons safflower oil
1 cup chopped dates
2 tablespoons pure maple syrup
¼ teaspoon pure vanilla extract
½ teaspoon pure almond extract
¾ cup whole spelt flour
½ teaspoon baking soda
⅛ teaspoon sea salt
½ cup unsweetened carob chips
¼ cup rolled oats
½ cup raisins

1. Preheat the oven to 375°F.

2. Push the carrot through the juicer. Set aside 2 tablespoons of the pulp.

3. In the oven, toast the pecans and almonds on an ungreased 11-by-15-inch cookie sheet for approximately 10 minutes, stirring occasionally. (Be careful not to let them burn, as this causes bitterness.) Coarsely chop the nuts and set aside.

4. In a medium-sized mixing bowl, cream together the egg substitute, oil, dates, maple syrup, and vanilla and almond extracts. Add the carrot pulp and mix well.

5. In a small mixing bowl, sift together the flour, baking soda, and salt.

6. Add the flour mixture to the carrot mixture and blend well with a sturdy spoon. Stir in the nuts, carob chips, oats, and raisins.

7. Roll the dough into 1-inch balls. Place the balls on an un-greased 11-by-15-inch cookie sheet and bake for 15 minutes, or until the cookies are golden brown in color.

*Makes 16 Cookies*

# Living Protein Squares

### MEDJOOL DATE BOTTOM

> 1 cup sunflower seeds
>
> 1 cup medjool dates, pitted
>
> 1 cup peanut butter
>
> 1 banana, peeled and halved
>
> 1 teaspoon pure vanilla extract
>
> ¼ cup sifted carob powder
>
> 1 cup flaxseed meal
>
> 1 cup green vegetable powder
>
> 1 cup unsweetened coconut

### HONEY PEANUT TOPPING

> 1½ cups peanut butter
>
> 2 tablespoons honey

1. To prepare the Medjool Date Bottom, in a food processor, using the metal blade, process the sunflower seeds until powder-fine. Add the dates, peanut butter, banana, and vanilla extract. Process until well blended, about 2 minutes. Restart the food processor and add the carob powder, flaxseed meal, green vegetable powder, and coconut through the feed tube. Run until well combined, about 10 seconds.

2. With your hands, shape the date mixture into 1-inch squares (oil your hands slightly to prevent sticking). Place the squares on an 11-by-15-inch cookie sheet lined with parchment paper and set aside.

3. To prepare the Honey Peanut Topping, in a food processor, using the metal blade, process the peanut butter and honey until well blended.

4. With a knife, dot each square with a peanut honey top. Transfer the cookie sheet to the refrigerator and chill the squares on the top shelf for 1–2 hours, or until firm.

5. Serve accompanied by a cup of herbal tea.

*Makes 8 Servings*

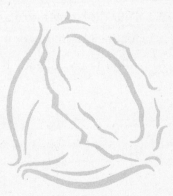

# Date Fudge Brownies

3 parsnips, cubed (½ cup pulp)

1 cup whole spelt flour

1 teaspoon baking powder

½ cup safflower oil

vegetarian egg substitute for 1 egg

¼ cup pure maple syrup

1 cup pure unsweetened cocoa powder (unsweetened
   carob powder may be substituted)

2½ cups chopped dates

1 teaspoon pure vanilla extract

½ cup ground unsalted almonds or almond butter

1 cup coarsely chopped unsalted walnuts

1. Preheat the oven to 350°F.

2. Push the parsnips through the juicer. Set aside ½ cup of the
   pulp.

3. In a small mixing bowl, sift together the flour and baking
   powder.

4. In a large mixing bowl, combine the oil, egg substitute, maple
   syrup, and cocoa. Add the parsnip pulp, dates, and vanilla
   extract and mix well. Add the flour mixture and mix again.
   Stir in the almonds and walnuts.

5. Pour the batter into a greased 10-inch square pan and bake
   for 30–40 minutes, or until firm.

6. Allow to cool slightly before cutting into 12 squares.

*Makes 12 Brownies*

# Pecan Chewies

6 parsnips, cubed (1 cup pulp)

1½ cups sweet rice syrup

½ cup raw almond butter

3 teaspoons pure almond extract

2 cups coarsely chopped unsalted pecans

1 cup blanched slivered almonds

1. Preheat the oven to 350°F.

2. Push the parsnips through the juicer. Set aside 1 cup of the pulp.

3. In a medium-sized mixing bowl, combine the sweet rice syrup, almond butter, and almond extract. Add the parsnip pulp, pecans, and almonds and mix well.

4. Pour the mixture into a greased 9-inch square baking dish and bake for 10 minutes, or until the nuts begin to turn light brown in color.

5. Cool for about 5 minutes before cutting into 6 squares.

*Makes 6 Chewies*

# Carob Power Brownies

½ cup sunflower seeds

1½ cups brown rice flour

½ cup carob powder

¾ teaspoon baking powder

¾ teaspoon ground nutmeg

¾ teaspoon sea salt

½ cup extra virgin olive oil

5 large bananas, peeled and coarsely chopped (about
2¼ cups)

1 cup bottled apple juice

1 cup bottled apricot juice

1 tablespoon honey

1½ teaspoons pure banana extract

1 cup walnuts, coarsely chopped

1 cup oat bran

½ cup plus 2 tablespoons rice bran

½ cup dairy-free carob chips

1.  Preheat oven to 350°F. Line two 12-well muffin tins with pa-per baking cups and set aside.

2.  Using a mini food processor or coffee grinder, process the sunflower seeds until powder-fine. Transfer to a mixing bowl and set aside.

3.  To make the brownies, in a large mixing bowl, sift together the flour, carob powder, baking powder, nutmeg, and salt. Whisk together until well mixed. Set aside.

4.  In a food processor, using a metal blade, combine the oil and bananas. Process until creamy, about 1 minute. Pour in the apple juice, apricot juice, honey, and banana extract. Process until well blended.

5. With a rubber spatula, gradually add the wet ingredients to the dry, making sure they are well blended before each addition. Scrape off any excess batter from the side of the bowl. Stir in the sunflower seed powder, walnuts, oat bran, rice bran, and carob chips until well mixed. Spoon the batter into the prepared muffin tins (the wells will be half full).

6. Bake in the middle level of the preheated oven for 35–40 minutes. For uniformity in baking, rotate the tin from front to back halfway through the baking period.

7. The brownies are done when a tester inserted in the center comes out clean. Remove the brownies from the oven and let cool completely, 15–20 minutes.

8. Serve with a glass of rice milk, soy milk, or nut milk.

*Makes 24 Brownies*

# Carob Fruit Bars

4 carrots, peeled, sliced lengthwise, tops removed
  (1 cup pulp)

¾ cup pure maple syrup

vegetarian egg substitute for 2 eggs

¼ cup light-colored honey (clover, tupelo, or wildflower)

1 teaspoon pure almond extract

½ teaspoon ground cinnamon

1 cup mashed bananas

1 cup unsweetened flaked coconut

¾ cup unsweetened carob chips

1 cup coarsely chopped unsalted pecans

¼ cup coarsely chopped unsalted macadamia nuts
  (pecans may be substituted)

2 tablespoons light oil

½ cup whole spelt flour

1.  Preheat the oven to 375°F.

2.  Push the carrots through the juicer. Set aside 1 cup of the
    pulp.

3.  In a medium-sized mixing bowl, whisk together the maple
    syrup, egg substitute, honey, almond extract, and cinnamon.
    Add the carrot pulp, bananas, coconut, carob chips, pecans,
    and macadamia nuts and stir well.

4.  In another medium-sized mixing bowl, combine the oil and
    flour and blend until a dough forms.

5.  Press the dough into a greased 9-by-12-inch baking dish. Pour
    the maple syrup mixture over the crust and bake for 15–20
    minutes.

6.  Allow to cool for 10 minutes before slicing into 12 bars.

*Makes 12 Bars*

# Grain Crispies Treats

1 parsnip, cubed (¼ cup pulp)

½ cup plus 2 tablespoons sweet rice syrup

½ cup peanut butter

1½ teaspoons pure almond extract

3 cups unsweetened grain flake cereal

¼ cup chopped dates

1. Push the parsnip through the juicer. Set aside ¼ cup of the pulp.

2. In a 2-quart saucepan, combine the rice syrup, peanut butter, and almond extract and bring to a simmer.

3. Remove the mixture from the heat and stir in the parsnip pulp, grain flakes, and dates, mixing together well.

4. Spoon the mixture into a greased 9-by-12-inch baking dish and press down firmly.

5. Cool completely before slicing into 9 bars.

*Makes 9 Bars*

# Banana Cocoa Sundae

2 peeled bananas, frozen (1 cup pulp)

2 tablespoons pure unsweetened cocoa powder

(unsweetened carob powder may be substituted)

2 tablespoons unsweetened flaked coconut

1. Push the frozen bananas through the juicer. Collect 1 cup of the pulp (mashed banana) in a small mixing bowl.

2. Add the cocoa to the pulp and mix together well.

3. Divide the mixture into two serving dishes, top with the coconut, and serve cold.

*Makes 2 Sundaes*

# Banana Nutmeg Sundae
# with Pineapple and Coconut

2 peeled bananas, frozen (1 cup pulp)

¼ cup fresh pineapple chunks

2 tablespoons unsweetened flaked coconut

¼ teaspoon ground nutmeg

1. Push the frozen bananas through the juicer. Collect 1 cup of the pulp (mashed banana).

2. Divide the banana pulp into two serving dishes, top with the remaining ingredients, and serve cold.

*Makes 2 Sundaes*

# Wonder Juice Float

1 medium kiwi, peeled and quartered

1 medium tangerine, peeled and quartered

2 medium oranges, peeled and quartered

¼ medium pineapple, rind removed, cored and cubed

¼ cup sparkling water

1 scoop soy ice cream (approx. ½ cup)

1. Push all the fruits through the juicer.

2. Add the sparkling water to the juice mixture in a tall glass and stir well.

3. Gently drop the scoop of soy ice cream into the juice mixture.

4. Serve immediately.

*Makes 2 Cups*

# Strawberry Chocolate Pops

2 peeled bananas, frozen (1 cup pulp)

4 cups honeydew melon chunks, rind removed (1⅓ cups juice)

1 cup frozen strawberries

1 tablespoon pure unsweetened cocoa powder
  (unsweetened carob powder may be substituted)

1 teaspoon pure lemon extract

1. Separately push the frozen bananas and the melon through the juicer. Set aside 1 cup of the banana pulp (mashed banana) and 1⅓ cups of the melon juice.

2. In a blender or food processor, combine the banana pulp and melon juice with the remaining ingredients and blend for 2 minutes, or until smooth.

3. Pour the mixture into six 5-ounce ice-pop molds and freeze for 3–4 hours, or until firm.

*Makes 6 Pops*

# Creamsicle Pops

8 oranges, peeled and quartered (2 cups juice)

1 cup plain soy yogurt

¼ cup unsweetened flaked coconut

¼ cup ground unsalted almonds or almond butter

1 tablespoon pure vanilla extract

1. Push the oranges through the juicer. Set aside 2 cups of the juice.

2. In a blender or food processor, combine the juice with the remaining ingredients and blend for 2 minutes, or until smooth.

3. Pour the mixture into six 5-ounce ice-pop molds and freeze for 3–4 hours, or until firm.

*Makes 6 Pops*

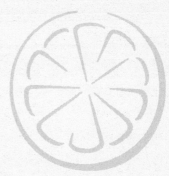

# Chocolate Coconut Pops

2 peeled bananas, frozen (1 cup pulp)

6 oranges, peeled and quartered (1½ cups juice)

½ cup plain soy yogurt

¼ cup unsweetened flaked coconut

2 tablespoons pure unsweetened cocoa powder
   (unsweetened carob powder may be substituted)

2 tablespoons ground unsalted pecans or pecan butter

2 teaspoons pure almond extract

1. Separately push the frozen bananas and the oranges through the juicer. Set aside 1 cup of the banana pulp (mashed banana) and 1½ cups of the orange juice.

2. In a blender or food processor, combine the banana pulp and orange juice with the remaining ingredients and blend for 2 minutes, or until smooth.

3. Pour the mixture into six 5-ounce ice-pop molds and freeze for 3–4 hours, or until firm.

*Makes 6 Pops*

# Raspberry Melon Pops

4 cups peeled watermelon chunks (1⅓ cups juice)

2 cups peeled honeydew melon chunks (⅔ cup juice)

2 lemons, peeled and quartered (¼ cup juice)

1½ cups frozen raspberries

2 teaspoons lemon extract

1. Separately push the watermelon, honeydew melon, and lemons through the juicer. Set aside 1⅓ cups of the watermelon juice, ⅔ cup of the honeydew melon juice, and ¼ cup of the lemon juice.

2. In a blender or food processor, combine the juices with the remaining ingredients and blend for 2 minutes, or until smooth.

3. Pour the mixture into six 5-ounce ice-pop molds and freeze for 3–4 hours, or until firm.

*Makes 6 Pops*

# Kiwi Lime Pops

    6 kiwis (1½ cups juice)

    4 cups peeled honeydew melon chunks (1⅓ cups juice)

    2 lemons, peeled and quartered (3 tablespoons juice)

    2 limes, peeled and quartered (3 tablespoons juice)

1.  Separately push the kiwis, melon, lemons, and limes through the juicer. Set aside 1½ cups of the kiwi juice, 1⅓ cups of the melon juice, 3 tablespoons of the lemon juice, and 3 tablespoons of the lime juice.

2.  In a small mixing bowl, combine the juices, mixing well with a spoon.

3.  Pour the mixture into six 5-ounce ice-pop molds and freeze for 3–4 hours, or until firm.

*Makes 6 Pops*


# Tropical Pops

    6 apples, cored and quartered (1½ cups juice)

    3 carrots, peeled, sliced lengthwise, tops removed
       (⅔ cup juice)

    2 peeled bananas, frozen (1 cup pulp)

    3 tablespoons chopped dates

    3 tablespoons unsweetened flaked coconut

    3 tablespoons ground unsalted almonds or almond butter

    1 teaspoon ground nutmeg

    1 teaspoon pure almond extract

1.  Separately push the apples, carrots, and frozen bananas through the juicer. Set aside 1½ cups of the apple juice, ⅔ cup of the carrot juice, and 1 cup of the banana pulp (mashed banana).

2.  In a blender or food processor, combine the juices and pulp with the remaining ingredients and blend for 2 minutes, or until smooth.

3.  Pour the mixture into six 5-ounce ice-pop molds and freeze for 3–4 hours, or until firm.

*Makes 6 Pops*

## Cherry Fruit Pops

1 lemon, peeled and quartered (2 tablespoons juice)
3 cups frozen pitted cherries (or any frozen berries)

1.  Push the lemons through the juicer. Set aside 2 tablespoons of the juice.

2.  In a blender or food processor, combine the lemon juice and cherries and blend for 2 minutes, or until smooth.

3.  Pour the mixture into six 5-ounce ice-pop molds and freeze for 3–4 hours, or until firm.

*Makes 6 Pops*

# Mango Fruit Pops

4 mangoes, peeled, pitted, and cubed (2 cups juice)

1½ pineapples, rind removed, cored and cubed (1½ cups juice)

1½ lemons, peeled and quartered (3 tablespoons juice)

1. Separately push the mangoes, pineapples, and lemons through the juicer. Set aside 2 cups of the mango juice, 1½ cups of the pineapple juice, and 3 tablespoons of the lemon juice.

2. In a small mixing bowl, combine the juices, mixing well with a spoon.

3. Pour the mixture into six 5-ounce ice-pop molds and freeze for 3–4 hours, or until firm.

*Makes 6 Pops*

# Lemon Lime Slush

1 eight-pound honeydew melon, rind removed, seeded and cut into 1-inch pieces

8 lemons, peeled and quartered

8 limes, peeled and quartered, plus 1 large lime, sliced into ¼-inch-thick half-moons, as garnish (optional)

1. Place a 4-cup-capacity liquid measuring cup under the juicer spout. Push the honeydew melon, lemons, and limes through the juicer. Reserve 1¼ cups juice and set aside in the refrigerator.

2. Pour the remaining juice into 4 ice cube trays and freeze for 1–2 hours, or until frozen.

3. Transfer the frozen cubes to a blender or food processor

and blend with the refrigerated juice until slush-like in consistency.

4.  Serve in tall glasses with straws and lime slices, if desired.

*Makes 10 Cups*

# Pineapple Orange Slush

4 large grapefruits, peeled and quartered

4 large oranges, peeled and quartered

½ large pineapple, rind removed, cored and cut into
1-inch pieces (about 4 cups)

16 nectarines, pitted and quartered

1.  Place a 4-cup-capacity liquid measuring cup under the juicer spout. Push the grapefruits, oranges, pineapple, and nectarines through the juicer. Reserve 1¼ cups juice and set aside in the refrigerator.

2.  Pour the remaining juice into 4 ice cube trays and freeze for 1–2 hours, or until frozen.

3.  Transfer the frozen cubes to a blender or food processor and blend with the refrigerated juice until slush-like in consistency.

4.  Serve in tall glasses with straws.

*Makes 12 Cups*

# The "Sublime" Water Slush

1 eight-pound watermelon, rind removed, cut into 1-inch
    cubes

3 large limes, peeled and quartered, plus 1 lime, sliced
    into ¼-inch-thick half-moons, as garnish (optional)

1.  Place a 4-cup-capacity liquid measuring cup under the juicer spout. Push the watermelon and 3 limes through the juicer. Reserve 1¼ cups juice and set aside in the refrigerator.

2.  Pour the remaining juice into 4 ice cube trays and freeze for 1–2 hours, or until frozen.

3.  Transfer the frozen cubes to a blender or food processor and blend with the refrigerated juice until slush-like in consistency.

4.  Serve in tall glasses with straws and lime slices, if desired.

*Makes 9–10 Cups*

# Tropical Ambrosia Pudding

1 tangerine, peeled and quartered (¼ cup juice)

1 mango, peeled, pitted, and cubed (½ cup juice)

¼ pineapple, rind removed, cored and cubed (¼ cup
    juice)

1½ cups silken tofu

¼ cup pure maple syrup

2 teaspoons pure almond extract

¼ teaspoon ground nutmeg

¾ cup mashed banana

3 tablespoons unsweetened flaked coconut

3 tablespoons raisins

3 tablespoons blanched slivered almonds

1. Separately push the tangerine, mango, and pineapple through the juicer. Set aside ¼ cup of the tangerine juice, ½ cup of the mango juice, and ¼ cup of the pineapple juice.

2. In a blender or food processor, combine the juices with the silken tofu and blend for 2–3 minutes, or until smooth.

3. Add the maple syrup, almond extract, and nutmeg and continue to blend.

4. Transfer the mixture to a small mixing bowl and stir in the banana, coconut, raisins, and almonds.

5. Chill for at least 1 hour before serving.

*Makes 2–4 Servings*

# Applesauce

5 apples, cored and quartered (1¼ cups juice and
   1 cup pulp)
1 tablespoon raisins
dash of ground cinnamon

1. Push the apples through the juicer. Set aside 1¼ cups of the juice and 1 cup of the pulp.

2. In a small saucepan, bring the apple juice to a boil over high heat.

3. Reduce the heat to medium-low and add the apple pulp, raisins, and cinnamon. Simmer for 5–10 minutes.

4. Serve hot or cold.

*Makes 1½ Cups*

# Strawberry Compote with Saffron Flowers

¼ pineapple, rind removed, cored and cubed
   (¼ cup juice)
1 teaspoon saffron threads
1 cup sliced strawberries
1 cup mashed banana
¼ teaspoon ground nutmeg

1.  Push the pineapple through the juicer. Set aside ¼ cup of the juice.

2.  In a small saucepan, combine the pineapple juice with the saffron threads. Cook over medium heat until the mixture comes to a simmer, and remove from the heat.

3.  In a blender or food processor, combine the pineapple mixture with the remaining ingredients and blend for 2 minutes, or until smooth. Transfer to a small bowl and chill for 1 hour.

4.  Serve cold over cake or ice cream.

*Makes 2 Cups*

# Granola Delight

    1 cup granola

    1 cup rice beverage

    ½ cup unsweetened carob chips

    1 cup vanilla soy ice cream

    2 bananas, peeled

    2 cups strawberries, hulled

    raspberry syrup

1. Blend all the ingredients except the raspberry syrup together in a blender until well combined.

2. Transfer blended mixture to dishes and drizzle desired amount of raspberry syrup over the top.

3. Serve immediately.

*Makes 5 Cups*


# Almond Joy with Soy

    4 ounces mineral water

    20 unsalted almonds

    2 dates, pitted

    2 ounces soft tofu

1. Blend all the ingredients together in a blender until smooth.

2. Serve immediately.

*Makes 1 Cup*

# Cherry Grape Kanten

6 cups bottled pineapple juice

¼ cup plus 2 tablespoons agar flakes (available at
health food stores)

8 medium ripe peaches, peeled, pitted, and sliced
(about 3 cups)

¼ large pineapple, rind removed, cored and cut into
1-inch pieces (about 2 cups)

2 cups seedless green grapes

2 twelve-ounce packages frozen pitted cherries

2 tablespoons freshly squeezed lemon juice

1. In a medium-sized saucepan, bring the pineapple juice to a
boil over high heat. Reduce heat to moderate and stir in the
agar.

2. Simmer uncovered, stirring occasionally, for 10 minutes, or
until the agar is completely dissolved.

3. In a large mixing bowl, toss the peaches, pineapple, grapes,
and cherries together with the lemon juice until well combined. Transfer to a 7-by-11-inch baking dish and pour in the
pineapple juice mixture. Let cool for 15 minutes; then refrigerate for 30–45 minutes, or until congealed.

4. Spoon into small bowls and serve.

*Makes 6–8 Servings*

# Healthy Fondue

2 peeled bananas, frozen

½ cup agar flakes

½ cup carob-flavored rice frozen dessert

1 pear, peeled, cored, and quartered

2½ cups pitted cherries

2 teaspoons vanilla powder

1. Blend the bananas, agar, and rice frozen dessert in a blender or food processor until smooth.

2. Push the pear and cherries through the juicer.

3. Add juice mixture and vanilla powder to the blended mixture and blend until well combined.

4. Transfer the mixture to a small pot and heat over low heat until warm. Use as a fondue dip for a variety of diced fruit or vegetables. In the alternative, freeze the blended mixture and serve frozen in a bowl.

*Makes 3 Cups*

# Cherry Yogurt Sauce

1 cup pitted cherries (½ cup juice and ½ cup pulp)

1 cup plain soy yogurt

1. Push the cherries through the juicer. Set aside ½ cup of the juice and ½ cup of the pulp.

2. In a small mixing bowl, combine the juice, pulp, and yogurt and stir until the mixture is well blended.

3. Serve cold with sliced fresh fruit, or spoon over cake.

*Variations:*

Substitute strawberries, blueberries, or raspberries for the cherries.

*Makes 2 Cups*

# Smooth Vanilla Sauce

2 cups vanilla-flavored soy milk

1 cup light coconut milk

1 vanilla bean, cut in half lengthwise (about 3.5 g)

2 teaspoons honey

¼ teaspoon sea salt

1 teaspoon pure vanilla extract

1. In a medium-sized saucepan, bring the soy milk and coconut milk to a simmer. With a wooden spoon, stir in the vanilla bean, honey, and salt. Reduce heat to low and simmer uncovered, stirring occasionally, for 25–30 minutes, or until the sauce reduces by two-thirds. Remove from the heat, then stir in the vanilla extract until well combined.

2. Serve hot or chilled over fresh fruit.

*Makes 3 Cups*

# Red Raspberry Coulis

2 cups frozen red raspberries

½ cup frozen orange juice concentrate

1. In a food processor, using the metal blade, combine the raspberries and concentrate. Process until creamy, about 3 minutes. Remove the blade and use a rubber spatula to scrape off any excess coulis remaining on the blade or processor.

2. Serve immediately.

*Makes 2½ Cups*

# Gary Null's Natural-Living Weight-Loss Tips

**1.** *Stop* being a couch potato.

 *Start* being more active.

 Exert more energy—use the stairs more, walk farther and for longer periods of time, and participate in more sports. Gradually establish a regular exercise routine involving running, cycling, or another aerobic activity.

**2.** *Stop* procrastinating.

 *Start* getting things done.

 Finishing things that you have been putting off will make you feel better about yourself and help keep your mind off food. Take up a cause, hobby, project, or even a new romance that renews your interest in life and makes you want to get up in the morning.

**3.** *Stop* being passive.

   *Start* taking charge of your life.

   Using food for comfort and reward is inappropriate, and soothing your sorrows and frustrations with fattening foods may actually deepen your depression. Instead of overeating, analyze what is bothering you and take steps to eliminate the problem.

**4.** *Stop* punishing yourself with food.

   *Start* accepting yourself for what you are.

   Food is generally thought of as being pleasurable, but you might subconsciously be using food to punish yourself. Secretly, you may believe that you don't deserve to be pretty, popular, happy, or healthy. Stop being so hard on yourself and start loving who you really are.

**5.** *Stop* setting idealistic long-term goals that are difficult to achieve.

   *Start* setting realistic short-term goals that you can reach.

   Whether the long-term goal is losing 10 pounds in one month or losing 100 pounds in one year, you are sure to run into temporary plateaus and disappointments—disappointments that could discourage you from continuing your efforts. It is better to set goals day by day or week by week. Then, if you make a mistake, you can forget it and move on to the next goal.

**6.** *Stop* isolating yourself.

> *Start* seeing people.

> Seeing people will help get your mind off food and end the depressing isolation you may impose on yourself when you feel fat and unattractive. Don't think you have to go it alone. If necessary, get help from a counselor or support group.

**7.** *Stop* thinking of yourself as dieting, starving, or deprived.

> *Start* realizing that you are permanently changing your life for the better.

> Generally, diets do not work. Most people regain lost weight in a dangerous diet yo-yo syndrome. Accept the fact that the healthy dietary changes you are making are permanent.

**8.** *Stop* putting food at the center of your life.

> *Start* expanding your life in new areas.

> Minimize the role of food in your social life. Join friends for sports or a movie rather than lunch. Find pleasurable activities other than meals to share with your family.

**9.** *Stop* thinking that you have to eat when and what the people around you are eating.

    *Start* eating only when you should eat and only what is good for you.

    If the three square meals a day your family eats are causing you unnecessary weight gain, don't eat them, *even if it means not eating with or cooking for your family.* You may need six small snacks a day to avoid the hunger pangs that sometimes plague meal-stretched stomachs.

**10.** *Stop* eating fats, animal products, and "empty calories" (sugar, refined carbohydrates, alcohol, etc.).

    *Start* eating more vegetables, fruits, and whole grains.

    Losing weight has less to do with counting calories than with eating right. Vegetables, fruits, and whole grains not only help you lose weight, but also make you healthier because of their high vitamin, mineral, and fiber content.

# Index